Develop Health and Inner Peace through Meditational Yoga

Jiwan D Jain

I would like to dedicate this book to Mr Narendra Modi, Prime Minister of India, whose action in getting the United Nations to declare 21st June as International Day of Yoga inspired me to write this book.

Foreword

My purpose in writing this book was two-fold:

1. To create a yoga practice that is suitable for people of all age groups and abilities, in particular, the growing number of people of advancing years who may find it difficult to carry out strenuous yoga poses.
2. To bring the principles of traditional yoga back into the practice, including elements of *pranayama*, meditation and breathing for relaxation.

Experience has shown me that carrying out yoga postures of a simpler nature, performed to the full ability of the practitioner, provides similar benefits to carrying out some of the more rigorous postures. What is important is that these are carried out correctly, with focus, and using breathing for the relaxation of the muscles that are being exercised and stretched. Introducing the meditational approach, which brings the mind into play and a visualisation of 'having a perfect body' during the course of the practice, enables the tremendous self-healing power of our bodies to enhance the health benefits of the postures.

My experience has also shown that *pranayamas* have a significant contribution to make to a yoga practice by improving the health and well-being of the internal organs.

I started yoga in India at the age of 10, but somewhat under duress. My father used to go to an ashram in Aravali Hills in Delhi to practise yoga. During the summer holidays, he would wake me up at 5 am to accompany him to the yoga class. Needless to say, I found every opportunity and all kinds of excuses to get out of this. However, in recollection, I feel that I inwardly enjoyed those classes as I could bend more, balance better and stretch into the postures more due to my age.

Many years later, I started going to yoga classes in the UK and immediately took a liking to them. This encouraged me to take up a diploma in teacher training with the British Wheel of Yoga. I taught yoga classes in the local gym and at some other institutions for a few years, and maintained my own practice at home. This is when I started to develop a routine that would cover exercising all parts of the body, including the joints and internal organs. I have always been interested in spiritualism and meditation, and meditational yoga was a culmination of all of this.

If you are starting this practice as a beginner, I very much hope you will find time to devote to understanding it, and will benefit from it by developing good health and inner peace. However, if you are already practising yoga, then I hope you will find some aspects of this book of use to add to your own practice.

With regular practice, you can build greater positivity and gradually eliminate negativity from your life. You will develop a mindset of living in the 'here and now', rather than regretting the past or worrying about the future. You will become more forgiving. With better control of your mind, you will find inner peace.

Throughout the structure of the book, I have kept the theme of meditational yoga in mind, and have started with a chapter on meditation that covers the types of meditation and the benefits of meditation, followed by a chapter covering the types of yoga and their benefits. The routine developed by me is in Chapter 4, to which readers may go to jump straight to the practice. At the end of the chapter on the practice (Chapter 4), I have added some advanced exercises that you can use as you progress further into your own practice. There are also details of some of the yoga *asanas* that are not included in the standard practice.

I have included a chapter on human anatomy (Chapter 6). As this book relates to the health of our bodies, I felt it appropriate to provide a quick reference point on how our bodies function. With my background in electronics engineering, it never ceases to amaze me what a marvel of engineering, science and creativity the human body is.

There is also a chapter on chakras (Chapter 5) as these form part of the progressive practices and will help to enhance the practitioner's spiritual experience.

Finally, there is a section describing the benefits of each of the *asanas* included in the practice (end of Chapter 4). Rather than disrupt the flow of the exercises by including these after the *asanas*, I felt it better to cover these in a separate place later on.

Please read this book in conjunction with the DVD on the practice of meditational yoga, which provides a demonstration of the complete practice.

Peace
Jiwan D Jain

Content List

1. Meditation

Meditation is a practice in which an individual operates or trains the mind, or induces a mode of consciousness.

Meditation has been practised in different cultures for centuries. The objective has remained the same, but the means, method and object of focus may have varied.

A. BUDDHIST MEDITATION

Buddha was a contemporary of Mahavir (the founder of the Jain religion), and followed the practices of Jainism in the beginning. However, he came to disagree with the concept of *atma* (soul) and that of reincarnation, and set out the ideology of Buddhism. Due to the patronage of King Ashoka, whose empire spread far and wide in the East, Buddhism also spread to Ceylon, Burma, Nepal, Tibet, Thailand, Korea, China and Japan.

Buddhist meditation techniques aim to develop *sati* (mindfulness), *samadhi* (concentration), *samatha* (equanimity), *abhijna* (transcendental powers) and *vipassana* (insight).

Two of the most popular techniques in use these days are the following:
- *Anapana sati* (mindfulness of breathing)
- *Vipassana* (seeing things as they really are)

1. Mindfulness of Breathing

Zen meditation is a form of mindfulness of breathing and is generally practised while sitting on the floor on a mat and cushion, with legs crossed in the lotus or half lotus position.

It can also be practised sitting on a chair, but the most important aspect is keeping your back, from the pelvis to the neck, completely straight. Your mouth is kept closed and your eyes are kept lowered, with your gaze resting on the ground about two or three feet in front of you.

Focus on your breath – focus all your attention on the movement of the breath going in and out through the nose. Sometimes counting the breaths in your mind is used as an aide to enhance focus.

In another form, known as *shikantaza* (just sitting), the practitioner does not use any specific object of meditation; rather, the practitioners remain as much as possible in the present moment, aware of and observing what passes through their minds and around them, without dwelling on anything in particular. It's a type of 'effortless presence' meditation.

2. Vipassana Meditation

Vipassana (seeing things as they really are) is the process of self- purification by self-observation.

Vipassana meditation focuses on insight or 'clear seeing', and has become one of the favourite forms of meditation in the West, popularised by S.N. Goenka.

Starting with focusing on the breath, the practice moves onto developing a clear insight on the bodily sensations and mental activity – just observing these but without any attachment.

As you focus on your breath, you notice that other perceptions and sensations start to appear: sounds, feelings in the body, emotions, etc. Simply notice these phenomena as they emerge in the field of awareness, and then return to the sensation of breathing. The attention is kept in the object of concentration (the breathing), while these other thoughts or sensations are there simply as 'background noise'.

3. Loving-kindness Meditation

This is a form of meditation that has been practised in Buddhism as a means of removing ill-will or hate. Once you are familiar with mindfulness of breathing and are practising it regularly, you can start practising loving-kindness meditation. First, you turn your attention to yourself and say to yourself phrases such as 'May I be well and happy. May I be peaceful and calm. May I be protected from dangers. May my mind be free from hatred. May my heart be filled with love. May I be well and happy.' Then, one by one, you think of a loved person; a neutral person – that is, someone you neither like nor dislike; and, finally, a disliked person, wishing each of them well as you do so.

Regular practice of loving-kindness meditation with the right attitude can bring about very positive changes in you. You will become more accepting and forgiving towards yourself. It also helps to increase the feelings towards your loved ones. It even encourages better relations with people you may have been indifferent to and uncaring towards. It also gradually eliminates the ill-will or resentment towards others. By including someone who is sick, unhappy or encountering difficulties in your meditation, it can sometimes help to improve their situation.

B. CHINESE MEDITATION

Meditation in China has been hugely influenced by Buddhist meditational techniques and some of these are still practised today.

Techniques developed specifically in China include the following:

1. Taoist Meditation

This has a long history, dating back 2,500 years, and is based on the Chinese philosophy of *Tao Te Ching*.

The chief characteristic of Taoist meditation is the generation, transformation and circulation of inner energy. The purpose is to quieten the body and mind, unify body and spirit, find inner peace, and harmonize with the Tao. Some styles of Taoist meditation are specifically focused on improving health and giving longevity.

There are two aspects that make this form of Chinese meditation different from others:

1. It emphasises living in harmony with nature – the way of nature. A person observes and reflects upon the things and phenomena around him or her, and learns to 'go with the flow'. It places importance on the Taoist concept of *we-wei*, which refers to non-action or action without the influence of its outcome.

2. It focuses on not only achieving a state of meditation but also achieving wisdom. A person develops an awareness that brings about knowledge, wisdom and greater control over his or her body. Unlike other

meditational techniques, the Chinese meditation guides the mind deliberately in a specific direction.

2. Qi Gong (Chi Kung) Meditation

This means 'life energy cultivation'. It is a holistic system of coordinated body postures, movement, breathing and meditation used for health, spirituality and martial-arts training.

The standing posture meditation technique, as it is known, is used to create and circulate *qi* (*chi* – life energy) around the body. The practice typically involves coordinating slow flowing movements; deep, rhythmic breathing; and a calm, meditative state of mind. The meditation has an important mental aspect to it in addition to its quiet, prominent, physical aspect; i.e. significant focus is required in bringing the mind's attention to ensure that the newly created *chi* is not lost.

Qi gong can be considered to be exercise as well as meditation. You will move every muscle, joint, bone and organ of the body in a slow and methodical way, and thereby develop and maintain flexibility.

This form of meditation helps to develop focus and concentration, and also builds the feeling of peace and harmony.

C. INDIAN MEDITATION

With its emphasis on the purpose of human life being 'to escape from a cycle of death and re-birth by attaining enlightenment', many Indian religions have meditation at the core of their practices. Indian scriptures show references to meditation going back thousands of years, using a number of different approaches to attain this goal.

In the *Yoga Sutras of Patanjali*, which describes an eight-fold path of yoga, the last three steps (*dharna, dhyana* and *samadhi*) underline the progressive states of meditation (please see Chapter 2 on yoga).

1. Jain Meditation

In Jainism, meditation is a core spiritual practice, one that Jains believe people have undertaken since the teaching of the *Tirthankara* Rishabha. All twenty-four *tirthankaras* practised deep meditation and attained enlightenment or *moksha*. They are all shown in meditative postures in the images or idols. Mahavira practised deep meditation for twelve years thereby attaining enlightenment.

There is another form of meditation lately in use in Jainism known as *preksha* meditation, which is the practice of purifying the emotions and consciousness (*chitta*), and realising one's own self. It helps in leading a peaceful life and is a system of meditation for attitudinal change, behavioural modification and the integrated development of personality.

The word '*preksha*' means 'to perceive carefully and profoundly'. In *preksha*, perception always means experience bereft of the duality of like and dislike, pleasure and pain. Impartiality and equanimity are synonymous with *preksha*. *Preksha* is impartial perception, where there is neither the emotion of attachment nor aversion, neither pleasure nor displeasure. Both these states of emotion are closely and carefully perceived but not experienced. And, because both are perceived from close quarters, it is not difficult to reject both of them and assume a neutral position. Thus, equanimity is essentially associated with *preksha* meditation.

2. Hindu Meditation

A number of practices have been used under Hindu meditation; some of the key ones are described as follows.

A. Mantra Meditation

A mantra is a syllable or word(s), usually without any particular meaning, that is repeated for the purpose of focusing your mind.

It is believed that the choice of word, and its correct pronunciation, is very important, due to the 'vibration' associated to the sound and meaning of the word. However, some feel that the mantra itself is only a tool to focus the mind, and the chosen word is completely irrelevant.

In addition to Hindu tradition, mantras are also used in Buddhist traditions, as well as in Jainism, Sikhism and Taoism (Chinese meditation). A more devotion-oriented practice of mantras is called *japa*, which consists of repeating sacred sounds (the name of God) with love.

It is usually practised sitting with the spine erect and eyes closed. The practitioner then repeats the mantra in his or her mind, silently (or vocally), over and over again during the whole session.

As you repeat the mantra, it creates a mental vibration that allows the mind to experience deeper levels of awareness. As you meditate, the mantra becomes increasingly abstract and indistinct, until you're finally led into the field of pure consciousness from which the vibration arose. Repetition of the mantra helps you disconnect from the thoughts filling your mind.

Some of the most well-known mantras from the Hindu and Buddhist traditions are as follows:

- Om (aum), ham, yam, ram, vam, lam (words denoting the symbols of the chakras or energy centres in the human body)
- Om arham
- So-ham
- Om namah shivaya

A practitioner will normally repeat the mantra a set number of times, traditionally 108 or 1,008, and beads are typically used for keeping count.

As the practice deepens, you may find that the mantra continues 'by itself', like the humming of the mind. Or the mantra may even disappear, and you are left in a state of deep inner peace.

People usually find that it is easier to focus with a mantra than with the breathing.

B. Transcendental Meditation

Transcendental meditation is a specific form of mantra meditation introduced by Maharishi Mahesh Yogi in 1955 in India and the West. In the late 1960s and early 1970s, the Maharishi achieved fame as the guru to The Beatles, The Beach Boys and other celebrities.

It is a widely practised form of meditation, with over 5 million practitioners worldwide, and there is a lot of scientific research, much sponsored by organisations, demonstrating the benefits of the practice.

To practise transcendental meditation it must be learned from one of their licensed instructors.

C. Yoga Meditations

Please also see chapter on yoga (Chapter 2).

In 'yogic meditation' the highest goal is spiritual purification and self-knowledge. It is part of an eight-fold path leading one to enlightenment.

There is a wide variety of practices for meditation in the yogic tradition.

D. Third-Eye Meditation

This focuses the attention on the 'spot between the eyebrows' (known as 'the third eye' or *ajna* chakra). The attention is constantly redirected to this point, as a means to silence the mind.

E. Chakra Meditation

The practitioner focuses on one of the seven chakras of the body (centres of energy), typically doing some visualisations and chanting a specific mantra for the chakra. Most commonly, it is done on the heart chakra, third-eye chakra or crown chakra.

There are other less-used forms of meditation, namely gazing meditation, *kundalini* meditation and sound meditation.

D. CHRISTIAN MEDITATION

'Meditation is a universal spiritual practice which guides us into the state of prayer, into the prayer of Christ. It brings us to silence, stillness and simplicity by a means that is itself silent, still and simple.' – Laurence Freeman, Your Daily Practice (cited in Giovanni, 2015)

The method involves the repetition of a single word faithfully and lovingly during the time of meditation. This is a very ancient Christian method of prayer that was recovered for modern Christians by the Benedictine monk John Main (1926–1982).

John Main recovered this way of bringing the mind to rest in the heart through his study of the teachings of the first Christian monks (the Desert Fathers) and of John Cassian (4th century AD). It is in the same tradition as *The Cloud of Unknowing*, written in England in the 14th century.

E. BENEFITS OF MEDITATION

Please refer to Giovanni (2015) for full references regarding the studies detailed below.

The National Institute of Health in US has now funded over 120 studies on the effect of meditation on various health issues, and the outcomes have been almost uniformly positive.

1. Stress Reduction

According to Dr Randy Zusman, MD, calming the mind during meditation, focusing attention on breathing and relaxing in a quiet state all help to reduce feelings of stress. A study conducted by Zusman finds that deep, controlled breathing also allows the body to produce increased levels of nitric oxide, a compound that helps open up constricted blood vessels and ultimately causes a reduction in blood pressure.

In another study it was found that people who practice 'mindful meditation' have a lower level of cortisol, which is a hormone produced in the adrenal glands whose primary function is to maintain energy levels and the body's functions when confronted with emotional and physical stress.

2. Heart Disease and Blood Pressure

A study published by the American Heart Association reports that participants who meditated throughout the study experienced a decrease in the thickness of their arterial walls, while those who did not meditate experienced no change to their arterial walls. The resulting decrease in arterial wall thickness translates into a lower risk of heart attack and stroke.

In March 2012, the *International Journal of Hypertension* found that meditation techniques appear to produce a small but meaningful reduction in blood pressure.

3. Decreased Muscle Tension

Drawing attention to different areas of the body by controlling breathing and calming the mind will help muscles relax. Progressive muscle relaxation can be used at the beginning of a meditation session to systematically tense and then relax muscles throughout your body.

4. Enhanced Immunity

According to a 2003 study published in *Psychosomatic Medicine*, meditation also has a demonstrably positive effect on the immune system and the brain.

A study from the University of Wisconsin also shows that meditation produces long-lasting beneficial changes in immune system function.

5. Mental Health

Mindfulness meditation has become an integral part of the treatment of various psychological disorders, such as anxiety, depression, post-traumatic stress, etc.

Research carried out at the Mayo Clinic indicates that meditation may also have a positive impact on a wide range of health conditions, including allergies, anxiety disorders, asthma, binge eating, depression, fatigue, heart disease, high blood pressure, pain, sleep problems, substance abuse and even cancer. According to experts, meditation is best used as a supplemental treatment in combination with other medical interventions.

6. Ageing

Research has also shown that meditation even slows the effects of the ageing process. People who meditate tend to look and feel much younger than their actual age.

7. Transcendental Meditation

Laboratory research into transcendental meditation reveals that during meditation the following physiological changes take place in the practitioner:

- Heartbeat and breathing rates slow down
- Oxygen consumption falls
- The blood lactate level drops
- Skin resistance to electric current increases fourfold, which is a sign of relaxation
- Electroencephalogram (EEG) readings of brain-wave patterns show increased alpha activity

F. HOW TO MEDITATE

1. Breathing Meditation

- Choose a quiet place to meditate and sit in a comfortable position. You can sit in *sukhasana*, in any other comfortable pose or even on a chair. The important thing is to keep your back straight and head upright.

- Gently close your eyes and bring the focus to your breath. Just breathe normally, and only observe and sense your breath flowing in and out. Also, remind yourself that with every breath you are inhaling the life-giving energy from the cosmos and with every outbreath you are expelling all impurities, all negative thoughts and all poisonous material from your body. Let your breathing grow gentler and deeper.

- Try and keep your mind's eye focused on the breath and bring it back every time it wanders off in another direction. As your mind settles down you may start feeling the senses pass signals to the brain – an itch or tingling in one part of your body. You should just observe these sensations without being distracted and allow them to pass. Gradually your distracting thoughts will subside, your mind will become still, and you will experience a sense of inner peace and relaxation.

- As you progress further in your practice, you can bring your mind's eye to focus at your 'eyebrow centre', and continue to breathe in and out. Stay in this position for 10 to 15 minutes and then gently come out.

Much of the stress and tension we normally experience comes from our minds, and many of the problems we experience, including ill health, are caused or aggravated by this stress. Just by doing breathing meditation for 10 to 15 minutes each day, you will be able to reduce this stress.

2. Meditation Using Chakras

Please refer to the chapter on chakras (Chapter 5).

- Start the chakra meditation in the same way as the breathing meditation. As your breathing settles down, take your focus to the root chakra (*muladhara* chakra) at the base of your spine, and visualise the breath flowing in and out of this chakra. Imagine red light glowing at this chakra. Feel yourself grounded and in contact with the Earth.

- Breathe in and out a few times, feeling the free flow of energy through the chakra before moving your focus to your sacral chakra (*svadhistana* chakra) located a couple of inches below your belly button. Imagine an orange light glowing at this chakra. Continue to breathe in and out, and visualise the chakra running freely, allowing the flow of energy within the body.

- Move your focus up to the solar plexus chakra (*manipura* chakra) at your naval centre, and visualise the energising breath flowing in and out. Imagine yellow light glowing at this chakra, and continue to breathe in and out a few times.

- Again, taking your mind's eye to focus on the next chakra, the heart chakra (*anahata* chakra) based at your heart centre. Imagine a green light flowing in and out of this chakra, and continue to breathe in and out a few more times.

- Move your focus to your throat centre (*vishuddhi* chakra) as you continue to breathe. Imagine blue light radiating from the chakra. Visualise the chakra running freely, allowing the smooth passage of energy through the body.

- Move up next to your eyebrow centre (*ajna* or third-eye chakra) – your vision centre where you see and resolve problems, and the centre of judgement. Imagine the chakra glowing in indigo light.
- Continue with a few breaths at this centre before moving to the crown chakra at the top of your head – your connection with the spiritual side. Imagine a violet light softly bathing your crown. Continue to breathe freely, and experience a feeling of peace, calm and tranquillity. Spend some time at this chakra before bringing your focus back to your breath and then to your physical body.
- Gently move your fingers, toes, arms and legs, bring the palms of your hands together and rub them gently. Place your warm palms on your eyes, gently slide your hands down and open your eyes.

2. Yoga

'Union of body and mind'

This can be seen as a set of physical, mental and spiritual practices to achieve the realisation of one's inner self.

The ancient scriptures of India show evidence of yoga practices going back to 2000 BC. One of these *Katha Upnishad* describes yoga as follows:

'When the senses are stilled, when the mind is at rest, when the intellect wavers not – then, say the wise, is reached the highest stage. This steady control of the senses and mind has been defined as Yoga.'

This may be seen as the prime aim of yoga, but a higher goal of yoga can be to attain *moksha* (liberation) or enlightenment, or *nirvana* or salvation, and end the cycle of death and re-birth, which is seen as the ultimate goal of human life in the Hindu, Jain and Buddhist philosophies.

A. PRINCIPLE PATHS OF YOGA

Indian scriptures define four principle paths of yoga as follows:

1. Jnana Yoga: Path of wisdom (or path of self-realisation)

This is the path of spiritual knowledge and wisdom, suited to the intellectual temperament, in which the intellect penetrates the veil of ignorance that prevents man from seeing his true self (*atma*). The practitioner usually studies with the aid of a guru.

2. Karma Yoga: Path of selfless action

Karma Yoga is the path of unselfish action. It teaches that a spiritual seeker should act according to *dharma*, without being attached to the fruits of their action or personal consequences.

3. Bhakti Yoga: Path of devotion and worship – the religious path

This is the yoga of strongly focused love, devotion and worship at its finest in love of the chosen god.

This form of yoga requires a complete surrender to the chosen deity/god. In turn, people practising this form of yoga become much more content and at peace with themselves as they come to believe that whatever happens in their lives has been granted to them by God, and must be their due and for their good.

4. Raja Yoga: Path of control of the mind

Raja Yoga is a systematic path of classical yoga leading one to the ultimate goal of human life – that of union with the Universal Spirit or *Param-atma* – thereby attaining salvation or nirvana.

The scriptures inform us that these four paths do not exist separately or in isolation. Each path is closely related to the other. When we think of God and are full of love for our fellow humans and for nature, we are Bhakti Yogis. When we stand by others and help we are Karma Yogis.

When we meditate and perform yoga practices, we are Raja Yogis. And, when we reflect upon the meaning of life and are explorers seeking truth and reality, we are Jnana Yogis.

B. PATANJALI'S EIGHT-FOLD PATH

However, from a Western perspective of yoga and for the purpose of this book, we will focus on Hatha Yoga, which forms part of Raja Yoga.

This system of yoga was first compiled by sage Patanjali between 5000 BC and AD 300. It is difficult to establish an exact time for this as for centuries the information was passed from teacher to disciple through word of mouth. In the later published work known as the *Yoga Sutras*, Patanjali describes an eight-fold path, detailing, step by step, how a person can find inner peace, health and knowledge through yoga. This eight-fold path is also known as Ashtanga Yoga and highlights a very scientific approach.

The eight steps (or limbs) prescribed by Patanjali are as follows:

- *Yamas:* (the five abstentions)
  - ✓ *Ahimsa* (non-violence, not harming other living beings)
  - ✓ *Satya* (truthfulness, non-falsehood)
  - ✓ *Asteya* (non-stealing)
  - ✓ *Brahamcharya* (celibacy, chastity or sexual restraint)
  - ✓ *Aparigraha (non-possessiveness)*

- *Niyamas:* (the five observances)

- ✓ *Shaucha* (purity/cleanliness of mind, speech and body)
- ✓ *Santosha* (contentment, acceptance of others and acceptance of one's circumstances)
- ✓ *Tapas* (persistent meditation, austerity and perseverance)
- ✓ *Swadhyaya* (self-reflection, introspection of one's own thoughts and actions)
- ✓ *Ishvar-pranidhan* (contemplation of the supreme being)

These two steps are aimed at preparing the body by developing the correct attitude and mental discipline for the following steps.

- ■ <u>*Asana* </u>: Posture

Asana is a generic term for a posture used in the practice of yoga, which is derived from the Sanskrit word for 'seat'. *Asanas* are aimed at increasing strength and flexibility in our body, improving balance and core strength, and bringing a sense of mindfulness into our everyday lives.

- ■ <u>*Pranayama:*</u>:

Control of the breath, from '*prana*' meaning 'life force or breath' and '*ayama*' meaning 'control'

Pranayamas are breathing exercises that clear the physical and emotional obstacles in our body to free the breath and so the flow of *prana* – life energy.

Although *pranayama*s form a limited part, if any, of modern-day yoga practice, their impact on revitalising the internal organs can be immense. I have therefore included a number of useful *pranayamas* in our practice below.

- *Pratyahara:* Freeing of the mind from the senses

- *Dharna:* Concentration and one-pointedness of the mind

- *Dhyana::* Meditation/contemplation

- *Samadhi:* State of super consciousness, oneness with the subject of meditation

The aforementioned systematic approach puts yoga in the category of science. The aim of yoga is to clear the mind, improve the quality of the mind and understand the reality of the mind.

The *asanas* keep your body healthy, strong and limber/supple.

Thousands of years ago, yogis in India had already completed an in-depth study of the nature of *healthy* minds and worked out how to achieve self-realisation. These techniques are sound and time tested, and hold truer than ever today.

C. YOGA IN THE WEST

Yoga gained prominence in the West in the late 19th century, following its introduction by Swami Vivekananda in the US. In the 1980s, yoga became extremely popular across the Western world as a system of physical exercises suitable for all age groups.

Over the years, a number of variations of yoga have evolved in the West to suit the different requirements and tastes of the practitioner, be it physical fitness and maintenance of a healthy body, for developing strength and suppleness in the muscles, or to attain a calm and peaceful mind. There are also some amended versions created to suit the needs of certain groups of people, e.g. to cater for the physically challenged or for pregnant women. The following lists some prominent types that have emerged over the years (in alphabetical order):

1. Anusara Yoga

Developed by American yogi John Friend in 1997, it is based on the intrinsic goodness in human beings. Anusara Yoga enables individuals to express themselves to their fullest ability through their yoga postures.

2. Ashtanga Yoga

Ashtanga Yoga is based on ancient yoga teachings. It is a rigorous form of yoga that follows a specific sequence of postures and is a physically demanding practice. Practitioners move rapidly from one *asana* to another using the inhalation and exhalation of breath.

3. Bikram Yoga

Developed by Bikram Choudhury, it is a series of 26 *asanas* and *pranayamas*, which are performed in a room heated to approximately 40°C. It is a widely popular form of yoga in the West.

4. Hatha Yoga

Hatha is a combination of two words: '*ha*' meaning 'mind' and '*tha*' meaning 'the vital life force' (or *prana*). Historically, Hatha Yoga meant the union of *pranic* and mental forces, which results in an awakening of higher consciousness.

It was believed that, before taking to the practices of meditation, you must first purify the body and its elements. In ancient times, the practice of *asanas* in Hatha Yoga was a preparatory step for higher states of consciousness. With time, the real purpose of this great science has been altogether forgotten and Hatha Yoga has come to stand for a series of postures.

Nearly every type of yoga class taught in the West is Hatha Yoga.

5. Iyengar Yoga

This is a meticulous style of yoga named after its founder B.K.S. Iyengar. The practice focuses on developing a perfect alignment in a posture (*asana*) and uses a variety of props such as blocks, straps, harnesses, etc. to get the practitioners more perfectly into the required positions. In his book *Light on Yoga*, Iyengar writes '*It contains the complete technique of 200 asanas with 592 photographs from which the asanas can be mastered; and it also covers* bandha, kriya *and* pranayama *with a further 5 photographs.*'

6. Sivananda Yoga

This is a relaxed form of yoga practice that will typically consist of 12 basic asanas, which are preceded and ended with *shavasana* and *surya namaskar*. Its theme is a five-point approach of proper breathing, relaxation, diet, exercise and positive thinking to produce a healthy yogic lifestyle.

7. Viniyasa Yoga

This is an active and athletic style of yoga adapted from the Ashtanga system to appeal to aerobic-minded practitioners. It is known for its fluid movement from pose to pose, linking breath to the movements. It is quite an intensive form of practice.

As we can see, a number of styles have come into being, but whether these all follow the values and spirit of yoga is perhaps debatable.

D. RESURGENCE IN INDIA

There has also been a resurgence of yoga in India in the last 10 years, with the appearance of Swami Ramdev. He has made it popular with the masses by holding large yoga sessions with demonstrations of simple-to-follow yoga *asanas* as well as *pranayamas*. A large number of people claim to have benefitted from these sessions in the form of curing many of their chronic illnesses.

In an interview with Swami Ramdev, he explained that he has included a greater element of *pranayamas* in the routine that he teaches as these are more effective in improving the health of the inner organs.

E. INTERNATIONAL DAY OF YOGA

On 11 December 2014, the 193-member United Nations (UN) General Assembly approved, by consensus, a resolution establishing 21 June as the International Day of Yoga. This came about in response to a call by Indian Prime Minister Narendra Modi during his address to the UN General Assembly on 27 September 2014.

The first International Day of Yoga was observed world over on 21 June 2015. About 35,000 people, including Indian Prime Minister Narendra Modi and a large number of dignitaries, performed 21 yoga *asanas* for 35 minutes at Rajpath in New Delhi, India. The day devoted to yoga was observed by millions across the world. The event at Rajpath established two Guinness World Records: the largest yoga class (with 35,985 people) and the record for the most nationalities (84) participating in it.

This day has since been celebrated every year by a large number of countries around the world by holding a day of yoga.

F. BENEFITS OF YOGA

Healing is a core element of both yoga philosophy and yoga practice. It is something we all aspire to, even if we do not always realise it—we all want to be healthy physically, mentally and emotionally.

Most people come to yoga because of some kind of discomfort, ailment or pain. Often, it's a physical ailment, such as arthritis or a stiff lower back. It could be that our muscles are tight due to stress or a sedentary lifestyle, and we want to increase our range of motion and become more flexible. Or it could be pain of a deeper nature - chronic stress, past trauma, a failed relationship or the realisation of the effects of ageing.

However, medical research in recent years has uncovered many physical and mental benefits offered by yoga, corroborating the experiences of millions of practitioners. A small sampling of research shows the following benefits of yoga:

- It is beneficial for physical fitness, musculoskeletal functionality and cardiovascular health.

- It is beneficial in the management of diabetes, respiratory disorders, hypertension, hypotension and many lifestyle-related disorders.
- It helps to reduce depression, fatigue, anxiety disorders and stress.
- It regulates menopausal symptoms.
- In essence, it is a process of creating a body and mind that leads to an exuberant and fulfilling life.

At the end of Chapter 4, I have included the specific benefits that can be achieved from each of the activities that are included in the practice.

In an article in the *Yoga Journal*, Aug 2007, Dr Timothy McCall, MD, lists the following 38 benefits of yoga:

1. Improves our flexibility
2. Builds muscle strength
3. Perfects our posture
4. Prevents cartilage and joint breakdown
5. Protects our spine
6. Betters our bone health
7. Increases our blood flow
8. Drains our lymph glands and boosts immunity
9. Ups our heart rate
10. Drops our blood pressure
11. Regulates our adrenal glands
12. Makes us happier
13. Founds a healthy lifestyle
14. Lowers blood sugar
15. Helps us focus
16. Relaxes our system
17. Improves our balance
18. Maintains our nervous system
19. Releases tension in our limbs

20. Helps us sleep more deeply
21. Boosts our immune system's functionality
22. Gives our lungs room to breathe
23. Prevents inflammatory bowel syndrome (IBS) and other digestive problems
24. Gives us peace of mind
25. Increases our self-esteem
26. Eases our pain
27. Gives us inner strength
28. Connects us with guidance
29. Helps keep us drug free
30. Builds awareness for transformation
31. Benefits our relationships
32. Uses sounds to soothe our sinuses
33. Guides our body's healing in our mind's eye
34. Keeps allergies and viruses at bay
35. Helps us serve others
36. Encourages self-care
37. Supports your connective tissue
38. Uses the placebo effect, to effect change

Please see the following link to read the full article:
https://www.yogajournal.com/lifestyle/count-yoga-38-ways-yoga-keeps-fit

3. Breathing

'Breath – the very essence of life'

Breathing is the only activity that enables our body to take in the life-giving energy from the cosmos during inhalation, and allows us to expel the impurities and poisonous matter from our body during exhalation.

Most of us take shallow breaths, which are restricted to upper chest. On average, a shallow breather inhales about 500 cc of air, but the deep breather can draw in about 4,000 cc of air. Thus, deep breathing takes in eight times as much air as shallow breathing, which fails to adequately aerate the alveoli of the lungs (see section on the respiratory system). But even in a deep breather the vital capacity is only 75% of total lung capacity.

The air we inhale is composed of 21% oxygen (O_2)(this percentage also includes carbon dioxide [CO_2]) and 79% of nitrogen (N_2). The oxygen to nitrogen balance is maintained, and we cannot increase the percentage of oxygen, but we can improve the ability of the lungs to take in more air and to process air.

If we look at a breakdown of the oxygen and carbon dioxide, the air we inhale is composed of 20.95% oxygen, 0.05% carbon dioxide and 79% nitrogen, and the exhaled air contains 16.5% oxygen, 4% carbon dioxide and 79.5% nitrogen.

All of the aforementioned breakdown points to a higher amount of oxygen being made available to our body and a higher amount of carbon dioxide being expelled from the body by regular deep breathing.

A. FULL YOGA BREATH

It is a well-known fact that we generally leave a large amount of stale air in our lungs when we breathe out. By practising the full yoga breath we can improve upon this and enable the lungs to work to a fuller capacity. The full yoga breath relies on abdominal breathing – how a baby breathes when he/she is born. Also see the chapter on the practice (Chapter 4).

B. FOCUSED BREATHING (WITH VISUALISATION)

In 'meditational yoga' breathing takes on an altogether different dimension. Focused breathing allows us to direct the breath to any part of the body. By visualising the breath flowing into a part of the body, we help direct the oxygen to the cells in that part and energise and invigorate those cells. Also, during the *asanas*, by directing the breath to the muscles that are being stretched we help to relax those muscles and relax into the posture. Focused breathing can also be used to relax tension from any part of the body.

C. PRANAYAMA

The yogic science of breath control should be at the very heart of a Hatha Yoga practice. Breathing exercises are essential for the purification, whereby the cells and nerve channels are cleansed and made ready for the advanced control of subtle energies. *Pranayamas* not only increase the capacity of the lungs but, by improving the efficiency of the respiratory system, they enhance the absorption of oxygen into our blood stream.

D. THE IMPORTANCE OF BREATH

Breath and how we breathe is an essential component of any yoga practice. A lot of research has been done on the effects of breath on our body.

In *Do, Breathe: Calm Your Mind*, Michael Townsend Williams writes:

'Awareness of our breath connects us to the way we move, the way we think and the way we feel. The way we breathe reflects the way we live. Animals that breathe quickly die early and the ones that breathe slowly live longer.'

Some additional opinions on the importance of breathing are as follows:

'If I had to limit my advice on healthier living to just one tip, it would be simply to learn how to breathe correctly.'

– Dr Andrew Weil

'Everything in the universe has a rhythm, from the movement of the planets to the beating of our hearts. Our breath is the connector with everything around us and with the universe.'

'Breathing creates a platform on which everything else – health, happiness, cognitive ability and elevated performance, success and influence – is built.'

– Dr Alan Watkins

'From our first breath to our last we breathe in and out somewhere in the region of 600 million times – taking in oxygen and breathing out carbon dioxide. Our breath is the crucial link between our mind and our body – the only system of our body which works both consciously and unconsciously. It effects how all our other internal systems work (digestion, immune system, heart, nerves, brain, etc.).

'Stress response: Our bodies are designed to maintain balance and any threats to this can trigger a flight or fight response which releases adrenaline and a myriad of other hormones to get us out of trouble.

'Relaxation response: Controlled deep breathing has been shown to produce the body's "relaxation response". A number of hormones are released in the body which slow down our heart rate, relax muscles, calm our nerves and improve our immune system and digestion. In as little as one minute of focussed breathing it is possible to completely clear the bloodstream of the stress hormone cortisol.'

– Tony Schwartz,
Harvard Business Review

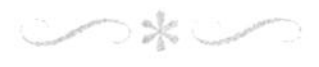

4. The Practice

I would like to start this chapter with a beautiful verse from the Indian scripture *Katha Upnishad*:

'But when a man has discrimination and his mind is controlled, his senses like the well-trained horses of a charioteer, lightly obey the reins... The man who has sound understanding for a charioteer and controlled mind for reins – he it is who reaches the end of the journey.'

Meditational yoga is focusing the mind intensely on your yoga practice, bringing it close to a state of meditation, and using your breath and the self-healing power of the mind to improve the health of the whole body. It helps to alleviate/eliminate aches and pains, and cure the body of many chronic diseases.

During practice, use your body as a guide to how far you go into a posture.

If you suffer from any ailments, it is prudent to seek advice from your doctor before taking up a new exercise regime. However, there are some specifics that I would like to include here for caution:

1. If you suffer from a coronary heart condition or have high blood pressure, please consult your medical adviser before continuing with the *kapalbhati* and *bahya pranayamas*. In any case, I would advise everyone to do *kapalbhati* gently and using small breaths.

2. If you have had back injury or are osteoporotic, you must do the back bends (bridge, cat, dog or cobra

poses) very gently initially, and increase the stretch over time and gradually as your body eases into the postures.

3. If you have knee problems or are unable to sit in *sukhasana,* you may sit on a chair to do the *pranayamas.*

So, what does meditational yoga bring to yoga practice? In the normal practice of yoga, one uses the breath to relax the muscles that are being stretched during a posture. In meditational yoga, you first still the mind and bring it to focus internally, connecting with your body and what is happening within the body during your yoga practice. A combination of mental visualisation and focused breathing exercises all internal organs, joints and muscles, and energises them.

Visualise your perfect and healthy body throughout your yoga practice.

In the next section is a demonstration of a simple routine that I have developed, which can be followed by young and old alike, and provides the same benefits as some of the more strenuous postures may do.

Yoga practice should be carried out on empty stomach, ideally in the morning after your daily cleaning routine, or at any time during the day after a gap of at least two hours following a meal.

You should choose a place that offers calm and quiet and is at a comfortable temperature. You could place a mat on the floor or use the carpet or any suitable floor covering.

You should wear clothes that are comfortable and allow free movement during the *asanas.*

I have produced this sequence of *asanas, pranayamas* and limbering exercises to enable the whole body, internal organs and joints of the body to be exercised. The purpose is to make it suitable for people of all abilities and all age groups.

Since you are reading this, I imagine that either you are a beginner and your aim is to improve your health and peace of mind. You can certainly achieve these by regular practice as shown in the following. Or, if you are a regular practitioner of yoga, you may be able to take elements of this sequence to add to your routine or to add some *asanas* from your current routine to this sequence as appropriate.

A. FULL YOGA BREATH

At the start of the practice, I want to introduce the full yoga breath that you will be using during most of your practice.

- Lie on your back (in *shavasana*) with your feet about 12–15 inches apart and rolled to the side, and your hands resting slightly away from the body with the palms facing up to the ceiling.
- Lift your head up slightly and, extending the neck, bring the head gently back down to the floor.

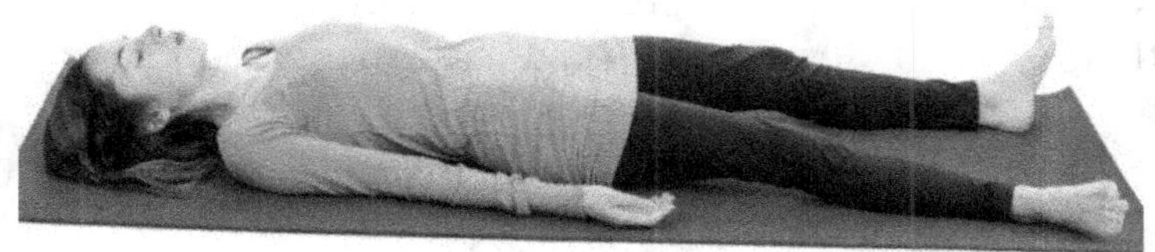

- Bring your focus to your breath, which should be a gentle rhythmic breath flowing in and out.
- Once settled, place both your palms on the top of your abdomen (belly) with the tips of your fingers touching. Focus on breathing into your abdomen and feel your fingers parting from each other as you inhale. Gently exhale and repeat the process a few times.
- Place your palms above your rib cage and, as you breathe into your abdomen and extend the breath further, you should find the fingers of your hands parting from each other. Repeat this a few times.
- Finally, place the palms of your hands on your upper chest with the tips of your fingers resting on your collar bone. As you breathe into your abdomen, then into the middle of your chest and, finally, into the top of your chest, filling up your lungs to their full capacity, you should feel your collar bones lifting towards your ears.
- As you breathe out, you breathe out gently from the top of your chest first, then the middle of your chest and finally from your abdomen – emptying your lungs completely.

This is the full yoga breath.

Let us remind ourselves that, every time we inhale, we breathe in the life-giving energy from the cosmos and, as we breathe out, we expel all the impurities, all negative thoughts and all poisonous material from our bodies.

B. THE PRACTICE

- Start your practice by lying on a mat on your back, in *shavasana*, with your feet spread slightly and palms facing towards the ceiling.
- Bring your focus to your breath, allowing it to become relaxed and extending it into the full yoga breath. Use the full yoga breath during relaxation and wherever possible during the practice.

1. Relaxation and Meditative State

- Focus on your left leg and visualise your breath flowing in from the tips of your toes, up your ankle, through your calf muscles, through your knee joint, via your thigh muscles and, finally, to your hip joint as you reach the end of the inhalation.
- As you breathe out, visualise it traversing down from your hip joint, all the way to the tips of your toes. Repeat that one more time feeling the whole of your left leg relax completely.
- Move your focus to your right leg next, repeating same steps (but for your right leg) and relaxing all the muscles in your right leg.
- Next, move your mind's eye to focus on your left arm, visualising your breath flowing in from the tips of your fingers, up your lower arm, through your elbow, along your upper arm and, finally, ending at your shoulder joint.
- Exhale gently, feeling your breath flow down from your shoulder joint all the way to the tips of your fingers. Repeat it one more time.
- Repeat the same twice for the right arm.

- Bring your mind to focus on your lower back next, letting your breath flow in and out of your lower back and relaxing the muscles in that region. Repeat this one more time.
- Repeat the same twice, focusing on the middle of your back, your upper back, the back of your neck, the back of your head, the top of your head, your forehead and face, the front of your neck, your chest, your abdomen and, finally, your heart; visualise and feel the muscles relax in the region that you are working on.
- The whole body should feel totally relaxed and your mind should be focused on your gentle breath flowing in and out.

  By bringing your mind into a state of meditation, you are able to communicate with your body and observe what is happening within as you conduct your *asana* and *pranayamas.*

From now on, keep your thoughts totally on your practice and your focus on your breath.

- Bring your attention back to your physical body, and bring your feet together and your arms close to your body with palms facing down.
- As you take the next in-breath, slowly raise your hands up towards the ceiling and keep them going till they come to rest on the floor above your head as you come to the end of the inhalation. As you start the exhalation, gently bring your hands back down to the sides of your body. Repeat this five to six times and when your hands next come to rest on the floor above your head, keep them there.

- Let your breath flow out gently and, as you take the next in-breath, stretch your hands upwards and your toes downwards, feeling the stretch running all the way from the tips of your fingers to the tips of your toes. Also, feel the stretch and a gentle tightening of the frontal muscles of your abdomen. This helps to flatten the stomach. Hold the stretch for as long is comfortable while breathing in and out gently.
- Let go of the stretch and relax.
- Stretch down from your heels next, enabling the stretch and extension of the muscles in your back. Hold the stretch for a while and then relax.
- Fold your knees and bring your arms around your knees, pressing the legs down towards the chest. If it is comfortable, raise your head gently towards your knees and hold for 10 seconds. (**Do not do this if you suffer from spondylitis or any neck problems.**) Gently bring your head down, release your arms and straighten out your legs.
- Take two to three relaxing breaths.

2. Bridge Pose

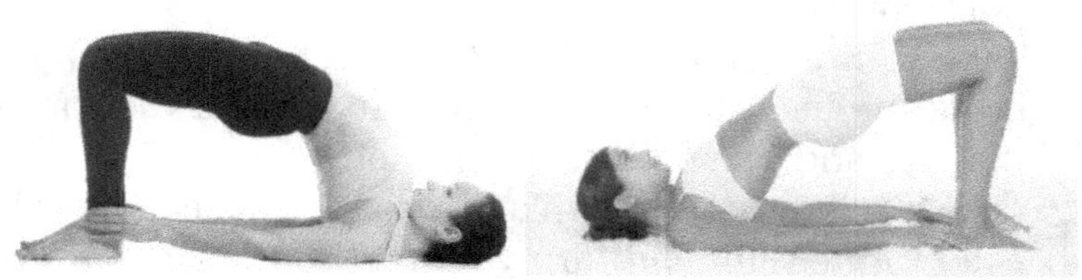

- Lie in *shavasana* and bring the soles of your feet to rest on the floor as close to your hips as possible.

- If you are a beginner, you may start by placing your hands by the sides of your body, with palms facing down.
- As you take the next in-breath, raise your pelvis towards the ceiling as far as you can, and, as you exhale gently, bring your pelvis down to the floor. Repeat this six times and on the last raise of your pelvis hold it there for as long as is comfortable, continuing to gently breathe in and out.
- As you grow in experience you will be able to hold your ankles with your hands and perform the *asana*, as shown in the picture at the beginning of the section.
- Lower your pelvis, straighten out your legs and relax.
- Fold your knees onto your chest and bring your arms around, hugging your legs to your chest, and gently rock from side to side to massage the muscles in your back.
- Unfold your arms, and as you unfold and straighten your legs keep rocking from side to side.
- Take a few breaths to relax as you come back into *shavasana.*

4. Spinal Twist

- Take your arms out to the sides with palms down, and bring the heel of your right foot to rest on the top of the first and second toes of your left foot.
- Take a full deep in-breath and, as you exhale, take your head to the right and turn your feet to the left, turning the pelvis with them. Try to keep your right shoulder in contact with the floor.
- Feel the stretch in the muscles in your pelvic area and upper thoracic area.

- Continue to breathe in and out, and relax those muscles, gently easing into the posture.
- Hold it for 10-15 seconds or three breaths, and then, as you exhale, bring your feet back to the centre and your head to the centre.
- Repeat the same steps by placing the heel of your left foot on the toes of your right, breathing in and turning your head to the left, and turning your feet and pelvis to the right as you breathe out.
- Hold the posture for three long yoga breaths while relaxing the stretched muscles and, finally, coming out of the posture as you exhale.
- Repeat the whole process once more on each side, allowing the stretch to extend a little bit and relaxing your muscles into the stretch.
- Come back to centre in *shavasana*, bring the soles of your feet to rest on the floor close to your hips and, as you exhale, take both knees to the left and your head to the right.
- Inhale, bringing your head and knees to the centre, and, as you exhale next time, take your knees to the right and your head to the left. Repeat the whole sequence 10 times on both sides.
- Bring your focus to your lower back and press it down towards the floor.
- Carry out a pelvic rotation on the floor by moving your pelvis upwards (towards the shoulders), to the right, downwards and towards the left. Continue this rotating movement 10 times, and then reverse the direction and repeat the rotation in the opposite direction 10 times.
- Fold your knees to your chest and place the palms of your hands on your knees.

- Rotate your hip joint in a circular movement by moving your knees apart, pushing them away from your body, bringing them together, bringing them towards your chest and, finally, moving them apart.
- Repeat this circular rotation 10 times in one direction, and then reverse the direction and repeat the rotation in the other direction 10 times.
- Straighten your legs and lie in *shavasana.*
- Take two to three breaths to relax.
- If you suffer from high blood pressure, you must avoid holding the in-breath.
- Take a deep breath in and, while holding the breath in, turn your body to the left, folding your knees slightly and placing your head on your folded left arm. Hold the breath for as long as is comfortable and gently exhale.
- Take another in-breath and, while holding the breath in, turn your body to the centre again. Hold the breath for some time and gently exhale.
- Take a deep breath in and repeat the same process to the right.
- Move back to the centre and then to the left once more. As you exhale and take the next in-breath, gently raise your body into a sitting position.

– bring yourself to believe in the recuperative power of your body.

We will now do some *pranayamas* that help to exercise the internal organs and rejuvenate them.

5. Kapalbhati Pranayama

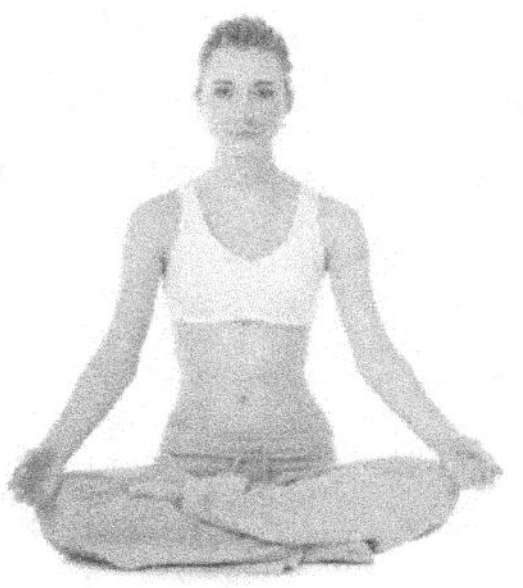

- Sit comfortably in *sukhasana* – legs crossed, back straight and upright, neck gently stretched, and head held upright. (If you are unable to sit cross-legged on the floor, you can also do this *pranayama* sitting on a chair.)
- Bring your hands into *gyan mudra* (with the tips of your thumb and first fingers touching, and your other three fingers straight), with the back of your hands resting on your knees.
- Keeping your back and head upright, take a breath in and, with an upward movement of your diaphragm, exhale the breath in a short burst (or you can visualise pulling the stomach muscles in to expel the air) and immediately let go, so that the natural recoil of the abdominal wall will bring in inspiration. Keep your shoulders relaxed and that they do not go up.
- Using 60 exhalations per minute (one per second), continue with these rhythmical exhalations for three minutes – exercising all the internal organs as you do so.
- Beginners may start the practice with a small number of breaths – say 10-20 – and repeat this three times

with a gap in between. Gradually extend into the full practice.

- After you have been practising this for a few weeks and feel comfortable with this process, you can move to the advanced stage of this as described in the advanced section.

6. Bahya Pranayama

- Continue sitting in *sukhasana* with your hands in *gyan mudra*; take a slow deep breath in; then, using the diaphragm and a little forcefully, exhale till the air is expelled from your lungs; and then pull your stomach in by lifting your diaphragm up.
- Hold this posture for as long as you can and then gently inhale.
- Relax and repeat this three times. Try to make sure that you keep your body tension-free while you are in the *pranayama*.
- Again, once you have been practising this for some time, you may extend into the next stage by applying the internal locks (see the advanced section).

You will now do some simple exercises to work on your leg muscles and joints.

- Sitting upright, stretch out your legs in front and place the palms of your hands by the sides of your body, keeping your back upright and relaxed.
- Stretch your legs by extending your toes outwards and hold for 10 seconds, then curl your toes inwards, stretch out from your heels and contract your thigh muscles – again hold for 10 seconds – and relax.
- Repeat this 10 times relaxing your muscles after they have been stretched fully.

- Move your attention next to the hip joint; fold your knees and bring the soles of your feet together, wrap your hands around your feet and bring your feet as close to your body as you can.
- Gently flex your knees up and down like a butterfly, exercising the hip joint.
- Do this 10–15 times.
- Take hold of your left leg in your hands just above the ankle and gently flick the foot in a rotating motion in a clockwise direction 10-15 times and then repeat the same in anticlockwise direction 10-15 times (exercising the ankle joint).
- Repeat for the other foot.

7. Anulom Vilom Pranayama

- Bring yourself to sit in *sukhasana* again.
- Keep your left hand on your knee in *gyan mudra* and bring the thumb of your right hand to rest gently on your right nostril, gently closing the nostril, and the rest of the fingers kept together but slightly away from the left nostril.
- Take a full deep breath in from the left nostril filling your lungs to their full capacity.
- At the end of the inhalation, remove your thumb from your right nostril and place the first finger of your right hand on your left nostril, closing the nostril, and after a momentary pause start a slow, gentle exhalation from the right nostril, expelling the air fully from your lungs.
- Start to inhale a full deep breath from your right nostril, filling your lungs to their full capacity, and again, after a brief pause, switch your thumb and first fingers to close the right nostril and open the left

nostril, and exhale slowly and gently to empty your lungs fully.

- Repeat this whole cycle 12 times and then come to rest in *sukhasana*.
- Relax with a few normal breaths before you start work on the joints in the arms.

You will now do some exercises to work on the joints in your arms:

- Sitting in *sukhasana*, place the palms of your hands on your knees and gently rotate them clockwise around the knees, at the same time rotate your shoulders, massaging your knees and flexing your shoulder joints.
- Repeat 10 times, and then change the direction of rotation and repeat in the anticlockwise direction 10 times.
- Next, place the tips of your fingers on your shoulders and make a circle with your elbows in a clockwise direction, repeating 10 times, and then reverse the direction and repeat 10 times.
- Take your arms above your head, fold your left arm and, holding the wrist of your left arm with your right hand behind your head, softly pull your wrist to the right, allowing a stretch in the muscles around your shoulder/upper back, and take three gentle breaths in and out, relaxing your stretched muscles.
- Let go of your left wrist and repeat the same movement on the other side.
- Repeat this exercise two more times.
- Stretch your arms above your head, intertwining your fingers and turning your palms towards the ceiling. Hold for a few breaths and relax.

- Place the palm of your right hand on the right side of your head and try to push your hand away using your neck muscles. Hold for two to three breaths and relax. Repeat on the other side.
- Intertwine your fingers, place the palms of your hands behind your head and press your head against your palms – hold for two to three breaths and repeat but with placing your palms at the front of your head.
- Sit in *sukhasana* and relax with a few normal breaths.

To work on the muscles in your legs:
- Lie down on your back, keeping your body straight and relaxed.
- Gently lift your right heel about 8-10 inches above the ground, keeping your knee straight, and hold this for a count of 10.
- Gently bring your heel down and repeat with the other leg.
- Repeat the whole exercise one more time, this time holding for a count of 50.
- Raise your right leg as high as you can and hold it there for a count of 10. Lower your leg and repeat on the other side.
- Repeat the whole exercise one more time, this time holding for a count of 50.
- Fold your knees and bring the soles of your feet to rest on the floor, slightly away from your hips.
- Straighten your right leg and lift it up as much as you can, again keeping your knee straight – you should feel the stretch in your hamstrings.
- Hold it for a count of 20 and relax the stretched muscles by breathing into them.

- Gently bring the leg down and repeat the movement with the other leg.

8. Cycling

- Lift your feet off the floor and make a cycling motion with your legs – one at a time, fold your leg up, stretching it up, keeping it straight, bringing it down and folding it back, and repeat this movement alternating between your legs. Repeat this 10 times.
- Reverse the direction of movement and again repeat 10 times.
- Bring your feet down and take a couple of breaths to relax.
- Carry out the same motion, but keeping both legs folded, and only lift the legs up, bring them down and folding them back – repeating five to six times.
- As your feet come to rest on the floor, bring your palms and wrap them around your knees, gently rock your body backwards and forwards, massaging the muscles in the whole of your back, and gently come into a sitting position.

8. Vajrasana (Thunderbolt Pose)

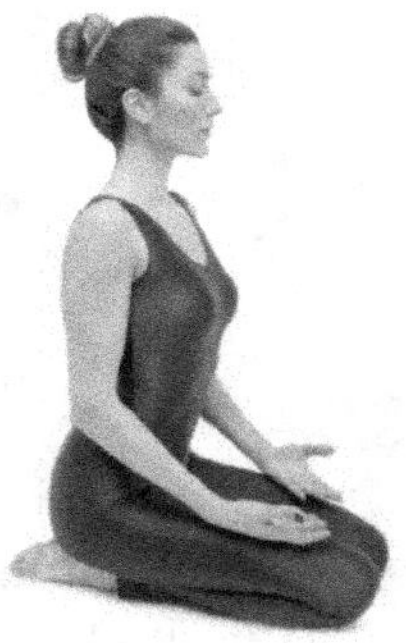

- Turn your body to face in the opposite direction and sit in *vajrasana* – sitting on folded knees, with the big toes of your feet touching and your heels spread apart; let your body sink onto your feet, and keep your back straight with your neck gently extended and head held upright.
- Relax your whole body and take a few deep in-breaths and out-breaths.
- Gently raise your hips a little, bring your toes together, spreading your heels, and rest back on your feet.
- Stretch your hands forwards, so that your arms are parallel to the floor with palms facing down.
- Take an in-breath, lift your body up into an upright position and then, as you exhale, bring your body down to rest back on your heels.
- Repeat this slowly six times and then lower your arms.
- If you are unable to sit in *vajrasana*, you may wish to do this sitting on a chair.

9. Cat Pose

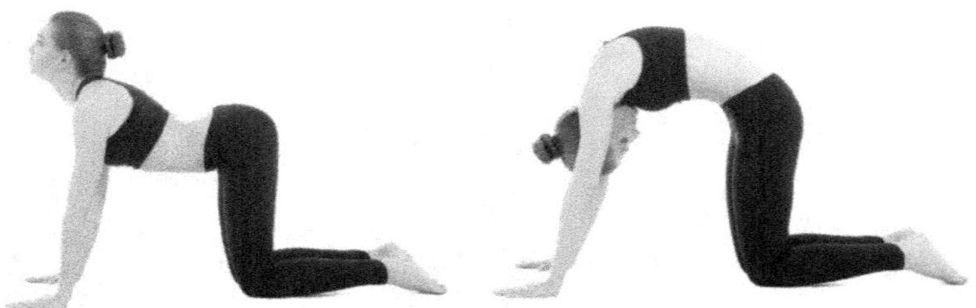

- Bring yourself to kneel on all fours, your legs about hip-width apart and your hands about shoulder width apart.
- As you take a deep breath in, gently lift your head up while making a concave arch in your spine.
- As you exhale, lower your head and arch your spine in the opposite direction (upwards).
- Feel the whole of your spine feeling the stretch and all vertebrae being exercised.
- Repeat this six times in line with your breathing.
- When you come to the middle next time, gently move to lie on the floor on your abdomen with your hands by the sides of your body.
- Relax your body with a few gentle breaths.

10. Bhujangasana (Cobra Pose)

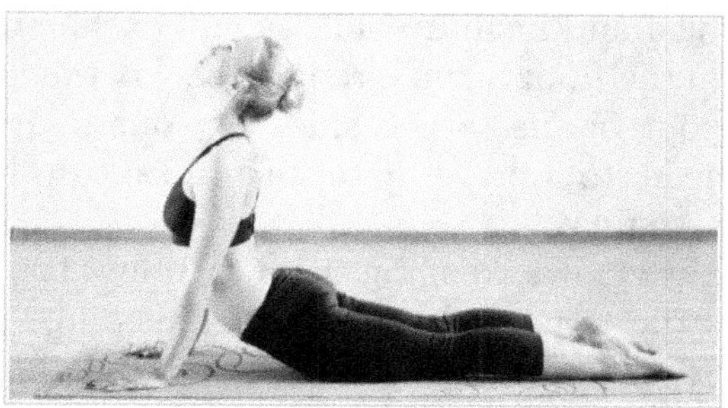

- Stretch out your hands, placing the palms of your hands on the floor above your head with your hands about shoulder width apart.
- Place your chin on the floor.
- Take an in-breath, raise your head and shoulders using the muscles in your upper back and hold it for a count of 10 while continuing to breathe normally.
- Gently lower your head to the floor.
- Lift your head, place your chin on the floor and bring your palms to rest by the sides of your face.
- As you take an in-breath, gently stretch out your neck, lift your head and raise it as high as you can, and look at a point in front of you. Keep your elbows soft and shoulders down.
- Continue breathing normally as you hold the stretch and, after three breaths, stretch your head backwards and look at the ceiling.
- Hold for another three normal breaths, bring your head to face the front, and then lower your head and shoulders gently to the floor.
- Turn your head to one side and take a couple of breaths to relax.

- Bring the palms of your hands to rest under your chin, one on top of the other. As you take a breath in, lift your chest and head up and, as you exhale, bring them down to the floor again – repeat this six times.
- Bring your hands to the sides of your body and turn your head to one side to relax. Take a few gentle breaths to relax.
- Fold your elbows, keeping them together; bring them to rest on the floor under your chin, keeping your hands upright; and bring your chin to rest on the palms of your hands.
- Fold your legs in turn, and try to touch your buttocks with the back of each heel. Repeat this on both sides six times.

11. Shalabhasana (Locust Pose)

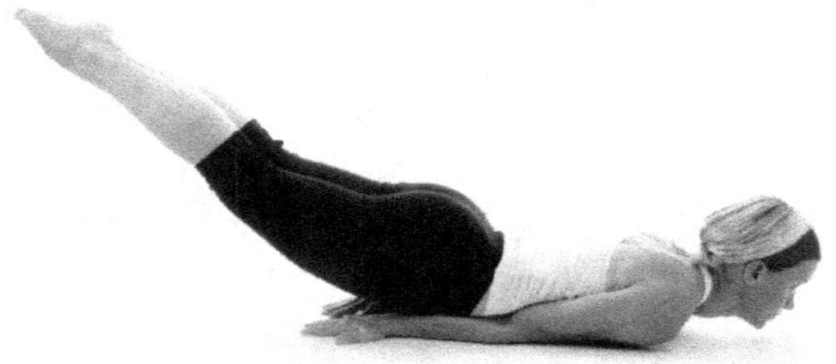

- Continue to lie on your abdomen, place the palms of your hands on top of one another and place them under your pelvis.
- Bring your chin to rest on the floor and gently lift your right leg up as much as you can, keeping your knee straight, and then hold the posture for a count of 10 while continuing to breath normally.
- Gently lower your leg, turn your head to the left and take a couple of breaths to relax.

- Bring your chin onto the floor and repeat with the left leg.
- Repeat the whole sequence one more time.
- Finally, bring your chin to the floor again, and this time lift both your legs up, and also raise your head and shoulders off the floor as much as you can. Hold for a count of 10, gently lower your body and relax with a few normal breaths.

12. Dog pose

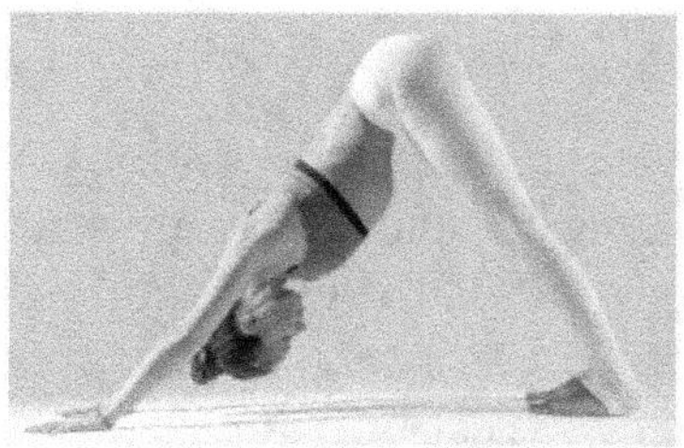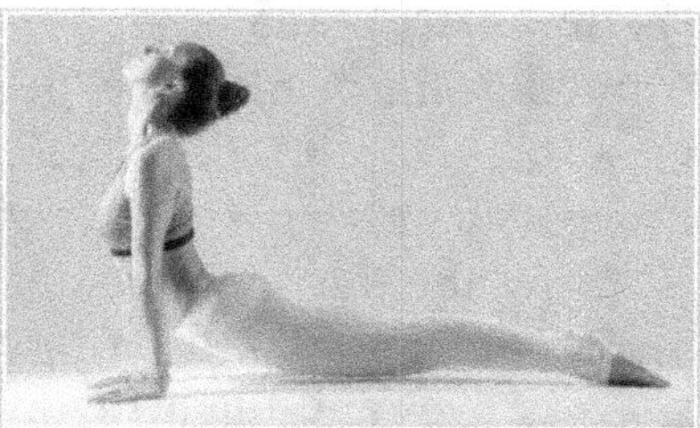

- Come to kneel on all fours, curling your toes in, and lift your pelvis up while straightening your legs, arms and upper body.
- Push your buttocks up towards the ceiling and towards the back of the body, creating a stretch in your legs.
- Feel the stretch in your whole body and relax into the stretch by breathing into the stretched muscles.
- Hold for as long as is comfortable and then, lowering your pelvis, lift your head up, bringing your chest into an upright position.
- Hold for a count of 10 and then go back into the pelvic lift, uncurl the toes and come to rest in the kneeling position; i.e. *vajrasana.*

- Stretch your arms out and place the palm of your left hand down and with your right hand forming a fist place it on top of the left.
- Bend from your pelvis, bring your chest down and bring your head to rest on top of your fist.
- Hold the posture for a count of 10 while breathing shallow breaths.
- Raise your body into *vajrasana* and relax.
- Take your body into *sukhasana*, ready for *bhramari pranayama*.

13. Bhramari Pranayama

From '*bhramari*', meaning 'bee'.

- Sitting comfortably in *sukhasana*, bring the thumbs of your hands to rest on your ears, closing your ears; bring the third fingers of your hands to rest on the tips of your nostrils, the first two fingers to rest gently on your eyes and the little fingers to rest on your lips.
- Take a deep breath in, press your third fingers to gently close your nostrils and exhale the air from your lungs, making a humming sound.
- Focus your mind's eye on the *ajna* chakra (the third eye – between your eyes at the centre of your forehead) feeling a vibration within.
- Repeat this three times.

This brings us to the end of the set exercises. At this point you have two choices. If you are a beginner or you feel you want to end the session here, you may continue and go into relaxation (as described in the next section). Otherwise, you can jump to *surya namaskar* and then come back to the relaxation – for this you need to come out of the meditative state.

C. RELAXATION

We will now completely relax the whole body by using a short form of *yoga nidra*.

- Lie on the mat in *shavasana* and start to feel your breath flowing in and out.
- Bring your mind's eye to focus on your breath and extend it into full yoga breath.
- Focus on your left leg and visualise your breath flowing in from the tips of your toes, up your ankle, through your calf muscles, through your knee joint, along your thigh muscles and, finally, to your hip joint as you reach the end of the inhalation.
- As you breathe out, visualise your breath traversing in the reverse order. Feel the whole of your left leg relax completely.
- Move your focus to your right leg next and repeat the same exercise, relaxing all the muscles in your right leg.
- Move your mind's eye to focus on your left arm, visualising your breath flowing in from the tips of your fingers, up your lower arm through your elbow, along your upper arm and, finally, ending at your shoulder joint.
- Exhale gently, feeling your breath flow down from your shoulder joint all the way to the tips of your fingers. Repeat the same for the right arm.
- Bring your mind to focus on your lower back, and let your breath flow in and out of your lower back, relaxing the muscles there.
- Repeat the same for the middle of your back, your upper back, the back of your neck, the back of your

head, the top of your head, your forehead and face, the front of your neck, your chest, your abdomen and, finally, your heart, and visualise and feel your heart muscles relax.

- Your whole body should feel totally relaxed and your mind should be focused on the deep gentle breath flowing in and out.

- Take your attention to your third eye – the point on your forehead between your eyes –and visualise your breath flowing in and out of your third eye. Continue this for a few breaths.

- Next, visualise a ball of white light floating in the air above your third eye and, as you take the next in-breath, visualise the white light entering your body – bringing the life-giving *prana* energy from the cosmos into your body.

- As you exhale, visualise the waste air coming out of your body, taking with it all impurities, all negative thoughts and poisonous matter from the body.

- As you continue to breathe in and out, visualise this white light is gradually spreading to all parts of your body, reaching all your cells, and revitalising and rejuvenating them. Keep this thought in mind and continue to breathe in and out for another three to five minutes.

- Gradually, you will feel your body becoming steady and relaxed, your mind becoming still, and you will experience a feeling of calm and inner peace.

- Gently bring your mind's eye to focus back on your physical body, and feel your legs, arms, spine, chest, abdomen and head.

- Give the fingers of your hands and the toes of your feet a quick shake.

- Rub your hands together, bring the palms of your hands to rest on your eyes and, after a few moments, remove your hands from your eyes.
- Turn your body to the left and gently come to a sitting position.

This is the end of the practice.

I realise that some of you may not find time in your daily schedule to do the complete routine. If that is the case, I would suggest that you split the routine as follows:

- <u>Day 1</u>: Carry out the first part of the practice up to and including the limbering exercises following the *anulom vilom pranayama*, and end (follow it) with relaxation.
- <u>Day 2</u>: Start with the relaxation and meditative state, then follow on from where you left off on Day 1 and carry on to the end, including *surya namaskar* and relaxation.

You can alternate these and also do the complete practice in between as time permits.

D. SURYA NAMASKAR (SUN SALUATION)

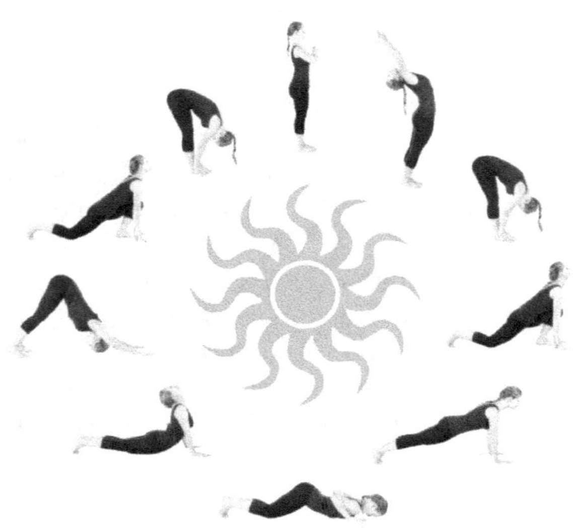

- Stand upright with your feet together, the palms of your hands together in front of your chest in '*namaste*', and your whole body feeling gently stretched upwards and relaxed.
- Breathe freely.
- While inhaling, open your arms with your palms facing forwards, and raise them upwards and back while lifting your head to look up at the sky (or ceiling).
- While exhaling, bend forwards from your hips, bring your hands down to touch the floor and place them by the sides of your feet (initially, you may need to bend your knees slightly).

- While inhaling, stretch your right leg back and go down on your right knee, at the same time lifting your head up.
- While holding your breath, straighten your left leg and bring your toes to rest by the side of your right toes, while straightening your left leg. Your body will be supported on your hands and toes.
- While exhaling, bend your arms, and lower your forehead, chest and knees to the floor. Keep your pelvis off the floor and your abdominal muscles pulled tight.
- While inhaling, straighten your arms, raise your upper body up and back to come into the *bhujangasana* (cobra) posture. Keep your elbows soft and shoulders down.
- While exhaling, lift your hips up, swing your head down between your arms and come into the 'dog with the head down' posture, with your legs straight at the knees and, if possible, your heels down with your feet flat on the floor.
- While inhaling, thrust your right leg forwards, at the same time bringing your left knee to touch the floor, and bring your right foot to rest on the floor by the side of your right hand, with your head and chest lifted up.
- While exhaling, bring your left foot forwards to place it by the side of your right foot and straighten your legs.
- While inhaling, straighten up, and raise your arms up and back as before.
- While exhaling, bring your arms back to the front in the starting position and breathe normally.

For greater benefit, you may repeat this three times.

With regular practice, you will build greater positivity and gradually eliminate negativity from your mind. You will develop a mindset of living in the 'here and now' rather than regretting the past or worrying about the future. You will become more forgiving. With better control of your mind, you will find inner peace.

E. ADVANCED EXERCISES

I have given some advanced exercises in this section that you can use as you progress further into your practice.

1. Kapalbhati Pranayama Using Chakras

- Sit comfortably in *sukhasana* – with your legs crossed, back straight and upright, neck gently stretched, and head held upright. Place your hands in *gyan mudra* (with the tips of your thumb and first fingers touching, and your other three fingers straight), with the backs of your hands resting on your knees.
- Take a breath in and with an upward movement of your diaphragm, exhale the breath in short bursts, keeping your focus on your *muladhara* chakra. Using 60 exhalations per minute (one per second), continue with these rhythmical exhalations for a count of 100.
- Move your focus to the *svadhistana* chakra and continue the exhalations for a count of 100.
- Step by step, move your focus to the *manipura* chakra, *anahata* chakra, *vishuddhi* chakra, *ajna* chakra and, finally, to the *sahasrara* chakra, and continue the gentle rhythmic exhalations for a count to 100 at every chakra.
- Stay in *sukhasana*, relax with few normal breaths, and enjoy the feeling of quiet and inner peace.

2. *Bahya Pranayama*

- Continue sitting in *sukhasana* with your hands in the same *gyan mudra* as before.
- Take a slow, deep breath in; then, a little forcefully, exhale till all the air is expelled from your lungs, and pull your stomach in by lifting your diaphragm up. Hold for as long as comfortable and then take a gentle breath in.
- Repeat the same one more time.
- Repeat the above but after expelling the air, focus on your diaphragm and move it up and down 20 times in slow rhythmic movements – massaging the organs within the stomach and chest area.
- Inhale and relax.
- Nauli: Repeat the deep inhalation and exhalation again. At the end of the exhalation, lift your diaphragm up as much as you can and, while you hold your diaphragm in this position, focus on your large intestines, and rotate them in a circular motion five times in one direction and then five times in the other direction.
- Inhale and relax.
- Lastly, repeat the deep inhalation and exhalation, try to touch your chin to your chest (applying the throat lock or *jalandhaa bandha*), lift the muscles of your diaphragm up (applying abdominal lock or *uddiyan bandha*) and also lift the muscles of your groin area, while squeezing your buttocks (applying *mooladhara bandha*). Hold this for as long as is comfortable.
- Release all the locks and breathe in slowly.
- Repeat this once more and relax.

3. Relaxation Using Chakras

- Sit comfortably in *sukhasana* and hold your hands in *gyan mudra* (i.e. with the tips of your thumb and first fingers pressing against one another, and the other three fingers held straight) and the backs of your hands resting on your knees.

- Keep your back, neck and head upright and relaxed, with your head looking straight in front.

- Close your eyes gently, bring your focus internally and feel the breath at the tip of the nose as you breathe in.

- Continue to breathe deep, long breaths, feeling each and every breath relaxing your body.

- Bring your mind's eye to focus on the *muladhara* chakra, which is based between your two genital organs, just in front of your anus (this is where your *kundalini* is based). Focusing on this chakra take a full yoga breath in and, as you exhale, visualise the energy from the chakra flowing into your body. Repeat this one more time.

- Move your focus to the *swadhistana* chakra, which is based just above your first genital organ, and, as you exhale, visualise the chakra running freely, allowing a smooth flow of energy. Repeat this one more time.

- Next take your focus to the *manipura* chakra, which is just behind your navel, and breathe into it, gently exhaling and visualising the free flow of energy through this chakra. Repeat this one more time.

- In turn, move your attention to the *anahata* chakra, which is based at your heart centre, then the *vishuddhi* chakra, which is based at the bottom of your throat, to the *ajna* chakra at the centre of your forehead and then, finally, to the *sahasrara* chakra at the top of your head, repeating the process of breathing in and out twice at each chakra.

- By going through all the chakras and experiencing the free flow of energy through the whole body, you bring your body to a state of peace and tranquillity.
- Stay with this for a few more breaths, then gently rub the palms of your hands together and bring your palms to rest on your eyes, gently open your eyes behind your closed fingers and spread your fingers to let the light in, and then remove your hands from your eyes.
- When you feel ready, you can raise yourself up.

F. ADDITIONAL STANDING ASANAS

1. Virbhadrasana (Warrior Poses 1 and 2)

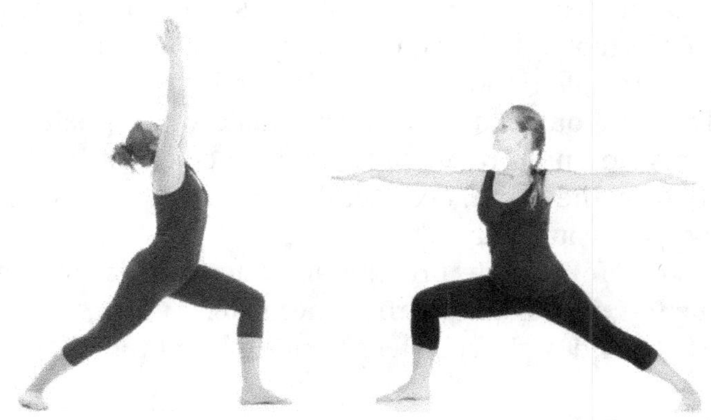

A. Warrior Pose 1
- Stand upright and take your feet about 3 ½ to 4 feet apart.

- Turn your left foot in 45° to the right and turn your right foot out 90° to the right. Your right heel should be in line with your left heel.
- Inhale and raise your arms upwards, parallel to each other and with your palms facing each other.
- As you exhale, turn your body to the right.
- Bend your right knee, moving it forwards so that your shin is perpendicular to the floor and your knee is above your right heel (make sure not to bend your knee too far to allow your thigh to be above your lower leg).
- Bring the palms of your hands together and stretch them upwards, feeling the stretch running up the back of your leg, across your belly and chest, and up into your arms.
- You can extend the pose by turning your head to look upwards at your hands.
- Breathe freely and hold the pose for as long as is comfortable, and gradually increase the duration until you are able to hold it for 30 seconds.
- To come out of the posture, inhale while raising your arms up and straightening your knee. Turn your body to face the front and gently drop your arms by the sides of your body.
- Take a few gentle breaths and then turn your feet to the left; repeat this to the other side.
- At the end, walk your feet to bring them together.

B. Warrior Pose 2

- Start the same as for Warrior Pose 1, but this time, rather than raising your arms above your head, raise them to the sides, parallel to the floor and with your palms facing down.

- Bend your right knee until it is over your heel and your lower leg is perpendicular to the floor.
- Stretch your right arm strongly to the right and your left arm to the left, in line with your shoulders.
- Turn your head to the right and gaze at your right hand.
- Hold the posture, and breathe freely and deeply. Gently return to the starting position and repeat on the other side.

2. Trikonasana

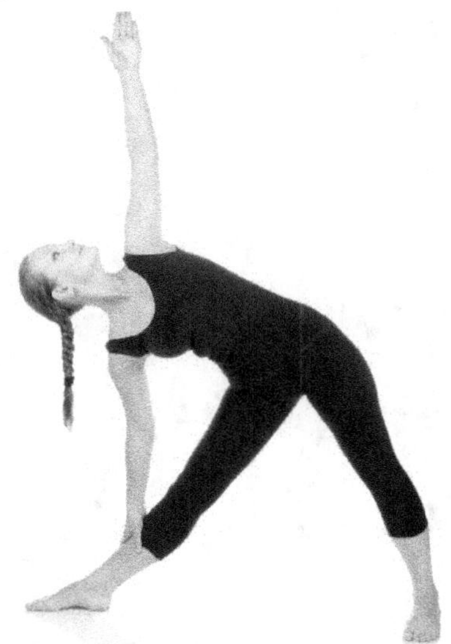

- Stand upright with your feet spread wide apart. Breathe in deeply, and extend your arms to the side and parallel to the floor with palms of your hands facing down.
- Keeping both arms and legs straight, bend from the waist to the right and place your right hand on the right leg sliding it down towards the ankle.

- As you progress, you may be able to bring your hand to rest on your foot or even on the floor by the side of your foot.
- Lift your left arm up, stretching upwards, and lift your head to look up at your left hand.
- Breathe freely and hold the posture for as long as is comfortable.
- Gently come out of the posture and repeat on the other side.

G. BENEFITS OF THE ACTIVITIES IN THE PRACTICE

Practice	Benefits
full yoga breath	It is considered to be a balancing *pranayama* as it balances the *vata*, *pitta* and *kapha* in the body. It is sometimes known as the three-part breath as it works with three different sections of the torso and engages all three lobes of the lungs.
shavasana	Helps to still and relax the body and mind; releases stress, fatigue and tension; and stimulates blood circulation.
bridge pose	Stretches the chest, neck, spine and hips. Strengthens the back and hamstrings. Improves digestion and the circulation of blood. Stimulates the lungs, thyroid glands and abdominal organs.
spinal twist	Aids digestion, relieves lower back pain, and strengthens the back muscles.
hip-joint rotation	Improves flexibility and

	strengthens the muscles around pelvic joint.
bahya pranayama	Helps to eliminate hernia, urinary and prostate problems, and removes gas and constipation problems.
kapalbhati pranayama	Helps to oxygenate the body and improves blood circulation; strengthens stomach/abdominal muscles; removes fat, giving a toned tummy; slows the ageing process; and affects the nervous system and sub-conscious mind.
anulom vilom pranayama	Purifies and balances the flow of energy in the body, increases oxygen supply throughout the body, improves concentration and decision-making ability, and brings a sense of calm and peacefulness to the body.
sukhasana	Helps to improve body posture, and stretches and lengthens the spine; calms the mind and brings a feeling of peacefulness by removing stress and anxiety.
cycling (*pada sanchalanasana* in Sanskrit)	Strengthens abdominal and lower back muscles, tones the thigh muscles, and improves hip- and knee-joint flexibility.

vajrasana	Stimulates digestion and aids liver function. It is the only pose that can be done on a full stomach.
cat pose	Stretches and strengthens the spine and neck; massages and stimulates the abdominal organs (kidneys, adrenal glands) and improves digestion; and improves the mobility of the hip joint.
bhujangasana (cobra pose)	Strengthens the muscles in the whole of the back, chest, stomach and pelvic areas. Follow this with the locust pose as a counter pose.
locust pose	Strengthens the muscles of the upper legs and lower back, strengthens the bladder, stimulates the stomach (relieves gas), and stretches the spine.
dog pose	Strengthens the hands, wrists, lower back, hamstrings, calves and Achilles tendon. Decreases back pain by strengthening the entire back and shoulder girdle. Brings blood flow back to the brain.
bhramari pranayama	Reduces fatigue and mental stress, improves concentration and provides a

feeling of happiness.

surya namaskar	Helps strengthen the muscles and joints of the whole body, and improves the flexibility of the spine; improves the digestive system; stimulates the nervous system; and helps to bring down the blood-sugar level.
trikonasana	Firms and tones the leg muscles, removes fat from the waistline, expands the chest, stretches the arms, shoulders and back, and massages the abdominal organs.
yoga nidra	Calms the nervous system; reduces stress, and promotes deep rest and relaxation; and helps to train the mind on the 'here and now'.
nauli	Strengthens the abdominal muscles, and massages the intestines and organs in the lower abdomen; regulates blood pressure; and helps with diabetes.
virbhadrasana	Limbers and strengthens the ankles, knees, hips and shoulders; tones the legs, hips, chest, back and neck; energises the whole body; expands the chest; and

loosens the hamstrings at the back of the legs.

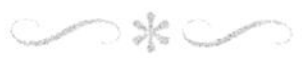

5. The Seven Chakras

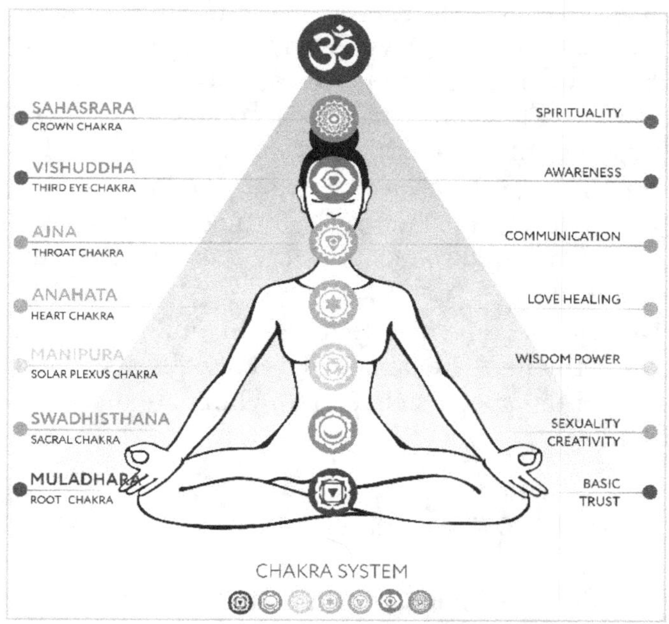

'Whenever I study the chakras, it never fails to amaze me of the perfection of our body and how well our body works in unison with nature and the world around us.'

Thousands of years ago, *rishis* (people of spiritual power) in India had experientially developed an advanced understanding of the human mind and body. A part of this knowledge was a system of *nadis* (astral tubes) that carried the *prana* within the body. Three key *nadis* are *sushmana*, *ida* and *pingla*. *Sushmana* is the main one of these and can be compared to the spinal cord. *Ida* and *pingla* are two entwined tubes that originate at the base of *sushmana*, and criss-cross at six points, which are the centres of six chakras.

The seven chakras (meaning 'wheel' in Sanskrit) describe the centres of energy within the human body that form the path for the flow of energy. Each of the chakras is associated with an organ, as well as with a human emotion or attribute. These also link to a colour, which indicates the frequency of energy that is transmitted by the chakra.

For the maintenance of a healthy body it is vital that energy is allowed to flow freely through these chakras, as these are connected to our physical, emotional, mental and spiritual levels.

We will be referring to these in our practice as we progress further. Advanced level Yogis use practices focused on the specific chakras to eliminate diseases from their bodies.

A. MULADHARA CHAKRA (ROOT CHAKRA)

From '*mula*', meaning 'root', and '*dhara*', meaning 'support'.

This represents our feeling of being grounded and physical survival; in this modern age, this also translates to financial and emotional security.

This is where *kundalini* energy is based.

- Location: At the base of the spine
- Colour: Red

- <u>Parts of the body that are affected</u>: Adrenal glands, kidneys, large intestines, spinal column, colon, legs and bones
- <u>Physical attributes</u>: Survival instincts and reproductive organs
- <u>Associated root word for meditation (chanting)</u>: Lam
- <u>Associated element</u>: Earth

B. SVADHISTANA CHAKRA (SACRAL CHAKRA)

From '*svadhistan*', meaning 'place of the self'.
This represents our identity as a human being and what we do with it.

- <u>Location</u>: Lower abdomen, 2 inches below the naval
- <u>Colour</u>: Orange
- <u>Parts of the body that are affected</u>: Lower abdomen, kidneys, bladder, circulatory system, and reproductive organs and glands
- <u>Physical attributes</u>: Tolerance, sexual and reproductive capacity, vitality, and pleasure
- <u>Root word</u>: Vam
- <u>Element</u>: Water

C. MANIPURA CHAKRA (SOLAR PLEXUS CHAKRA)

From '*manipura*', meaning lustrous gem.
This represents self-confidence, personal power and control in our lives.

- <u>Location</u>: Just above the naval centre

- <u>Colour</u>: Yellow
- <u>Parts of the body that are affected</u>: Pancreas, adrenals, stomach, liver, gallbladder, nervous system and muscles
- <u>Physical attributes</u>: Our sense of will power, autonomy and determination
- <u>Root word</u>: Ram
- <u>Element</u>: Fire

D. ANHATA CHAKRA (HEART CHAKRA)

From '*anhata*', meaning 'unhurt'.

This represents our ability to love, and express compassion and kindness.

- <u>Location</u>: Heart centre
- <u>Colour</u>: Bright green
- <u>Parts of the body that are affected</u>: Heart, thymus gland, circulatory system, arms, hands and lungs
- <u>Physical attributes</u>: Love, joy and inner peace
- <u>Root word</u>: Yam
- <u>Element</u>: Air

E. VISHUDDHI CHAKRA (THROAT CHAKRA)

From '*vishuddha*', meaning 'very pure'.
This represents our ability to communicate.

- <u>Location</u>: Throat centre
- <u>Colour</u>: Blue
- <u>Parts of the body that are affected</u>: Thyroid, parathyroid, hypothalamus, throat and mouth
- <u>Physical attributes</u>: Communication, self-expression, creativity, truth, logic and reason (judgement)

- Root word: Ham
- Element: Ether

F. AJNA CHAKRA (THIRD-EYE CHAKRA)

From '*ajna*', meaning 'beyond wisdom'.

Opens up your mind to information beyond the material world and the five senses.

- Location: Between the eyes on the forehead
- Colour: Indigo
- Parts of the body that are affected: Pituitary gland, pineal gland, nose and ears
- Physical attributes: Intuition; imagination; wisdom and the ability to think, analyse and make decisions; peace of mind; and forgiveness
- Root word: Om or aum

G. SAHASRARA CHAKRA (CROWN CHAKRA)

From '*sahasrara*', meaning 'thousand petaled'.

This represents pure consciousness energy and our ability to connect spiritually to the rest of the universe – a point of pure bliss.

- Location: Top of the crown
- Colour: Violet
- Parts of the body that are affected: Upper brain (cerebral cortex), central nervous system and the pituitary gland
- Physical attributes: Spiritual consciousness, connection to God, divine wisdom and pure bliss

6. Human Anatomy

A. THE HUMAN SKELETON

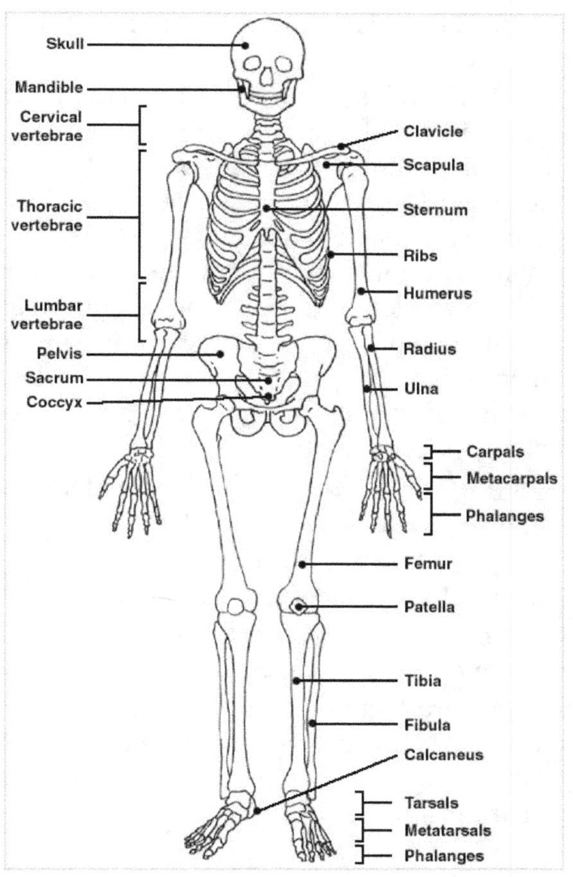

The **human skeleton** works as the internal framework of the body and is made up of mainly bones, cartilages and ligaments. It is composed of 270 bones at birth, but this reduces to around 206 by adulthood. There are also bands of fibrous connective tissue – the ligaments and the tendons – in intimate relationship with the parts of the skeleton.

1. Six Major Skeleton Functions

The skeleton serves six major functions in the human body:

- Support: It provides a framework to support the body and maintain its shape. The ribcage, costal cartilages and intercostal muscles provide support for the lungs. The floor for the pelvic structure is provided by the pelvis, associated ligaments and muscles.
- Movement: The joints between bones allow movement; some allow a wider range of movement than others, e.g. a ball-and-socket joint allows a greater range of movement than the pivot joint at the neck. Muscles, bones and joints provide the principal mechanics for movement, all coordinated by the nervous system.
- Protection: The skeleton helps to protect our many vital internal organs from being damaged:
  - ✓ The skull protects the brain.
  - ✓ The vertebrae protect the spinal cord.
  - ✓ The rib cage, spine and sternum protect the lungs, heart and major blood vessels.
- Blood cell production: The skeleton is the site of haematopoiesis, which is the development of blood cells that takes place in the bone marrow. In children, this occurs primarily in the marrow of the long bones,

such as the femur and tibia. In adults, it occurs mainly in the pelvis, cranium, vertebrae and sternum.

- <u>Storage</u>: The bones can store calcium and are involved in calcium metabolism, and bone marrow can store iron in ferritin and is involved in iron metabolism.
- <u>Endocrine regulation</u>: Bone cells release a hormone called osteocalcin, which contributes to the regulation of blood sugar (glucose) and fat deposition. Osteocalcin increases both the insulin secretion and sensitivity, in addition to boosting the number of insulin-producing cells and reducing stores of fat.

2. Principal Subdivisions

The human skeleton, can be described as consisting of two principal subdivisions, the **axial** and **appendicular** skeleton.

- The axial skeleton, consisting of 80 bones, is formed by the vertebral column (the spine), the rib cage and much of the skull. The upright posture of humans is maintained by the axial skeleton.
- The appendicular skeleton comprises of the pelvic (hip) and pectoral (shoulder) girdles and the bones and cartilages of the upper and lower limbs.

3. Vertebral Column

The vertebral column is not actually a column, but rather is a sort of spiral spring in the form of the letter S. A newborn child has a relatively straight backbone. The development of the curvatures occurs as the supporting functions of the vertebral column in humans (i.e. holding up the trunk, keeping the head erect, serving as an anchor for the extremities) are developed.

The S-curvature enables the vertebral column to absorb the shocks of walking on hard surfaces; a straight column would conduct the jarring shocks directly from the pelvic girdle to the head.

4. The Rib Cage

The rib cage, or thoracic basket, consists of the 12 thoracic (chest) vertebrae, the 24 ribs, and the breastbone or sternum.

When breathing in, through the action of a number of muscles, the rib cage, which is semi-rigid but expansile, increases its size. The pressure of the air in the lungs is thus reduced below that of the outside air, which moves into the lungs quickly to restore equilibrium. Expiration (breathing out) is a result of the relaxation of the respiratory muscles, the elastic recoil of the lungs, and the fibrous ligaments and tendons attached to the skeleton of the thorax.

A major respiratory muscle is the diaphragm, which separates the chest and abdomen, and has an extensive origin from the rib cage and the vertebral column. The configuration of the lower five ribs gives freedom for the expansion of the lower part of the rib cage and for the movements of the diaphragm.

5. Summary of the Main Bones of the Human Skeleton

- <u>Skull</u>: Cranium, mandible and maxilla
- <u>Shoulder girdle</u>: clavicle and scapula
- <u>Arm</u>: humerus, radius and ulna
- <u>Hand</u>: Carpals, metacarpals and phalanges
- <u>Chest</u>: Sternum and ribs
- <u>Spine</u>: Cervical area (top seven vertebrae), thoracic area (next twelve vertebrae), lumbar area (bottom five

vertebrae), sacrum (five fused or stuck together bones) and coccyx (the tiny bit at the bottom of the spine)

- <u>Pelvic girdle</u>: Ilium, pubis and ischium
- <u>Leg</u>: Femur, tibia and fibula
- <u>Ankle</u>: Talus and calcaneus (not shown in the previous diagram)
- <u>Foot</u>: Tarsals, metatarsals and phalanges.

B. THE HUMAN RESPIRATORY SYSTEM

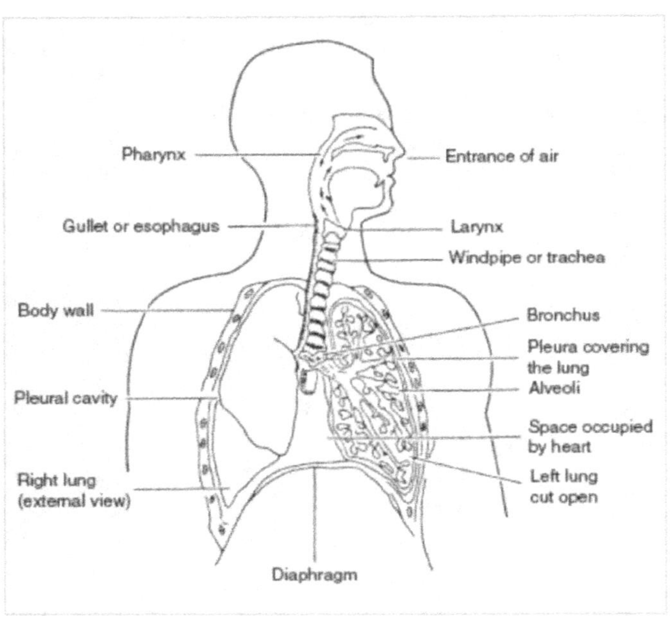

The essential features of respiration are (1) inhalation (inspiration), where oxygen is taken into the lungs, and thence to the blood and all the cells of the body; and (2) exhalation (expiration) where carbon dioxide, the main waste product of the cells, is expelled from the body. In addition, some water vapour is also excreted from the body and air supplied to the larynx for voice production.

The anatomy of the respiratory system is the respiratory tract, which is divided into an upper and a lower respiratory tract. The upper tract includes the nose, nasal cavities, sinuses, pharynx and the part of the larynx above the vocal folds. The lower tract includes the lower part of the larynx, the trachea, bronchi, bronchioles and the alveoli.

The preferred mode of breathing is through the nose, where the air is filtered by passing through the hair in the nostrils, also senses for chemicals of interest using the smell monitors, and the longer passage allows it to be warmed up and moistened. Breathing through the mouth uses a shorter passage and is therefore less efficient.

The lungs are covered by the pleura, which is a thin protective membrane, in two layers, one covering the lungs and the other lining the inner surface of the chest cavity, thereby allowing easy movement between the lungs and the thoracic cage. The right lung has three lobes and the left has two.

The diaphragm is an upwardly domed sheet of muscle that separates the thoracic cavity from the abdominal cavity. Inhalation at rest is primarily due to the contraction of the diaphragm.

In normal breathing, electrical messages are sent from the brain, via nerves, to the muscles of the ribcage and diaphragm. The contraction of these muscles causes the ribs to move outwards and the diaphragm to move downwards, increasing the size of the chest cavity and making the lungs expand. This creates a slight suction inside the lungs, and air rushes down to equalise the pressure. In breathing out, the electrical nerve messages stop, the muscles relax, and the natural elasticity of the lungs makes them shrink and expel the air.

Air entering the lungs consists of 20.95% oxygen, 79% nitrogen and 0.05% carbon dioxide. Air leaving the lungs contains 16% oxygen, 79% nitrogen and 4% carbon dioxide.

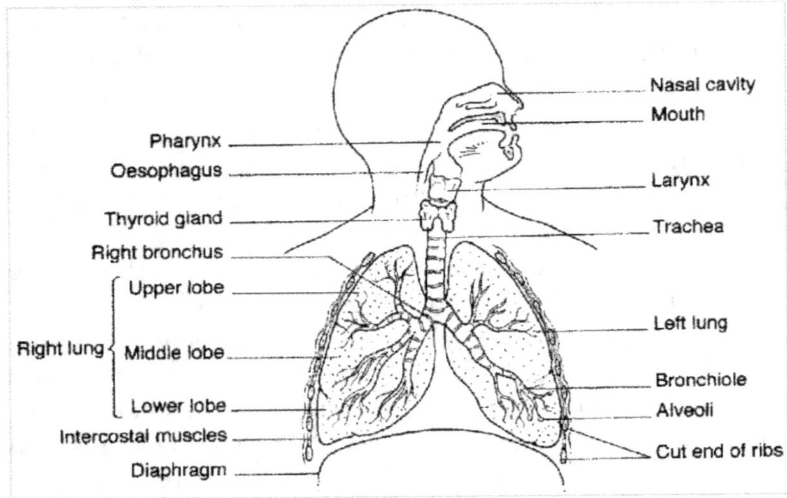

The trachea (also called the wind pipe) is guarded at its top by the epiglottis, so that food and drink are not inhaled.

The lower end of the trachea divides into two bronchi, each of which passes to the corresponding lung. From each main bronchus, numerous small bronchi are split off, like the branches of a tree, which further sub-divide, and the smallest of these tubes are called bronchioles. Each bronchiole terminates in an alveolus (air sac), which is made up of a number of air cells. These cells are surrounded by capillaries (small blood vessels), through the walls of which the interchange of gases takes place; i.e. oxygen flowing from the air sac into the blood and carbon dioxide passing from the blood into the air sacs.

Oxygen, having been passed into the tiny capillaries, is conveyed via the bloodstream to the heart, from where it is pumped to every part of the body.

Breathing is controlled as follows:

- <u>Automatic</u>: The nerve cells in the respiratory centre of the hind brain generate rhythmic electrical pulses, which act on the respiratory muscles as described previously.
- <u>Voluntary</u>: The cerebral motor cortex sends stronger electrical currents from the big nerve cells, which act on the respiratory centre and alter the rhythm as we wish, within certain limits.

C. THE DIGESTIVE SYSTEM

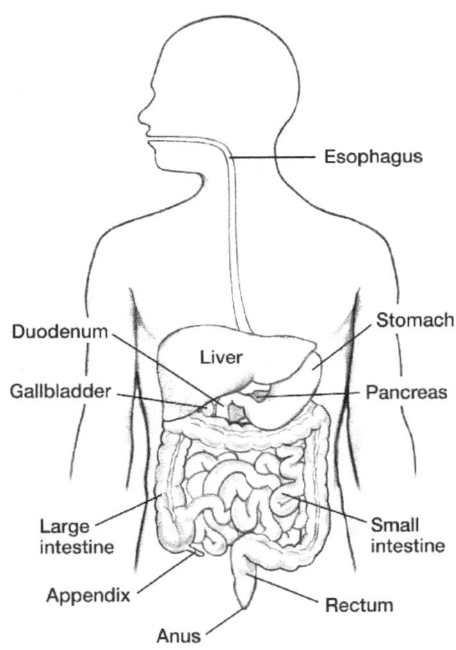

The **digestive system** carries out the vital role of processing the food and drink we consume by converting it into simple substances capable of being absorbed into the bloodstream – providing the energy we need to survive, and the nutrients we need for the growth, repair and maintenance of body tissues. It also deals with the waste by-products.

The digestive tract is a long, twisting tube that starts at the mouth and ends at the anus. It comprises a series of muscles in its wall, which coordinate the movement of food, and other cells in its lining that produce enzymes and hormones to aid in the breakdown of food. Along the way are three other organs that are needed for digestion: the liver, the gall bladder and the pancreas.

Other parts of the digestive system are described in the following sections.

1. The Mouth

Digestion begins in the mouth, where chewing begins the process of breaking the food down into pieces small enough to be digested. Saliva moistens the food to make it easier to swallow, and adds enzymes that help break down the starches into carbohydrates and also fats.

2. The Pharynx and Oesophagus

The pharynx (throat) is the portion of the digestive system that receives the food from the mouth in the form of bolus. Branching off the pharynx are the oesophagus, which carries food to the stomach, and the trachea (windpipe), which carries air to the lungs.

During the process of swallowing, muscles in the pharynx push the food into the oesophagus, at the same time closing off the trachea and preventing the food from entering the respiratory system.

The oesophagus, commonly known as the gullet, is an organ that consists of a muscular tube through which food passes from the pharynx to the stomach. Once in the oesophagus, the bolus travels down to the stomach via the rhythmic contraction and relaxation of the muscles, known as peristalsis.

3. The Stomach

The stomach is a major organ of the gastrointestinal (GI) tract and digestive system. It is a J-shaped organ joined to the oesophagus at its upper end and to the duodenum at its lower end.

The gastric acid (gastric juice) produced in the stomach plays a vital role in the digestive process, and mainly contains hydrochloric acid and sodium chloride. To prevent the corrosion of the stomach walls by the acid and strong enzymes produced for digestion, mucus is secreted by innumerable gastric glands in the stomach, which provides a slimy protective layer for the wall of the stomach.

At the same time as protein is being digested, mechanical churning occurs through the action of peristalsis, which are waves of muscular contractions that move along the stomach wall. This allows the mass of food to further mix with the digestive enzymes.

From the stomach, the food moves to the small intestine.

4. Small Intestine

Made up of three segments – the duodenum, jejunum and ileum – the small intestine also breaks down food using enzymes released by the pancreas and bile from the liver. Peristalsis is also at work here, moving food through the small intestine and mixing it with the digestive secretions from the pancreas and liver, including bile. The duodenum is largely responsible for continuing the process of nutrient breakdown or digestion, with the jejunum and ileum being mainly responsible for the absorption of nutrients into the bloodstream.

These processes are highly dependent on the activity of a large network of nerves, hormones and muscles.

While food is in the small intestine, nutrients are absorbed through the walls and into the bloodstream. What's leftover (the waste) moves into the large intestine (large bowel or colon).

Everything above the large intestine is called the upper GI tract. Everything below is called the lower GI tract.

5. The Colon, Rectum and Anus

The colon (large intestine) is a muscular tube that connects the small intestine to the rectum and is one and a half to two metres long. It is made up of the ascending (right) colon, the transverse (across) colon, the descending (left) colon and the sigmoid colon, which connects to the rectum. The appendix is a small tube attached to the ascending colon. The large intestine is a highly specialised organ that is responsible for processing waste and excreting it with ease.

It normally takes about 36 hours for stools to pass through the colon. The stools are mostly comprised of food debris and the bacteria that normally live in the colon. These bacteria perform several useful functions, such as synthesising various vitamins, processing waste products and food particles, and protecting against harmful bacteria. When the descending colon becomes full of stools it empties its contents into the rectum to begin the process of elimination.

The anus is the last part of the digestive system. It consists of the muscles that line the pelvis (pelvic-floor muscles) and two other muscles called anal sphincters (internal and external).

The pelvic-floor muscles create an angle between the rectum and the anus that stops stools from coming out when they are not supposed to. The anal sphincters provide fine control of the stools. The internal sphincter is always tight, except when stools enter the rectum. It keeps us continent (not releasing stools) when we are asleep or otherwise unaware of the presence of stools.

When we get an urge to defecate (go to the bathroom), we rely on our external sphincter to keep the stools in until we can get to the toilet.

6. Some Other Organs That Support the Digestive Process

- <u>Pancreas</u>: Among other functions, the pancreas is the chief factory for the digestive enzymes that are secreted into the duodenum, the first segment of the small intestine. These enzymes break down protein, fats and carbohydrates.
- <u>Liver</u>: The liver has multiple functions, but two of its main functions within the digestive system are to make and secrete an important substance called bile, and to process the blood coming from the small intestine containing the nutrients just absorbed. The liver purifies this blood of many impurities before it travels to the rest of the body.
- <u>Gall bladder</u>: The gall bladder is a storage sac for excess bile. Bile made in the liver travels to the small intestine via the bile ducts. If the intestine doesn't need it, the bile travels into the gallbladder, where it awaits the signal from the intestines that food is present. Bile serves two main purposes. Firstly, it helps absorb fats in the diet and, secondly, it carries waste from the liver that cannot go through the kidneys.

D. THE NERVOUS SYSTEM

The **nervous system** coordinates its actions by transmitting signals to and from different parts of our body. It does so using a complex network of nerves and cells that carry messages from the brain and spinal cord to various parts of the body, and vice versa. The nerves that transmit signals from the brain are called **motor** nerves, while those nerves that transmit information from the body to the central nervous system are called **sensory** nerves.

The nervous system can be defined in three parts:
1. The central nervous system (CNS); i.e. the brain and the spinal cord.
2. The peripheral nervous system (PNS), which forms the connection between the CNS and the organs and muscles of the body.
3. The autonomic (or involuntary) nervous system (ANS), which supplies the sympathetic and parasympathetic nerves.

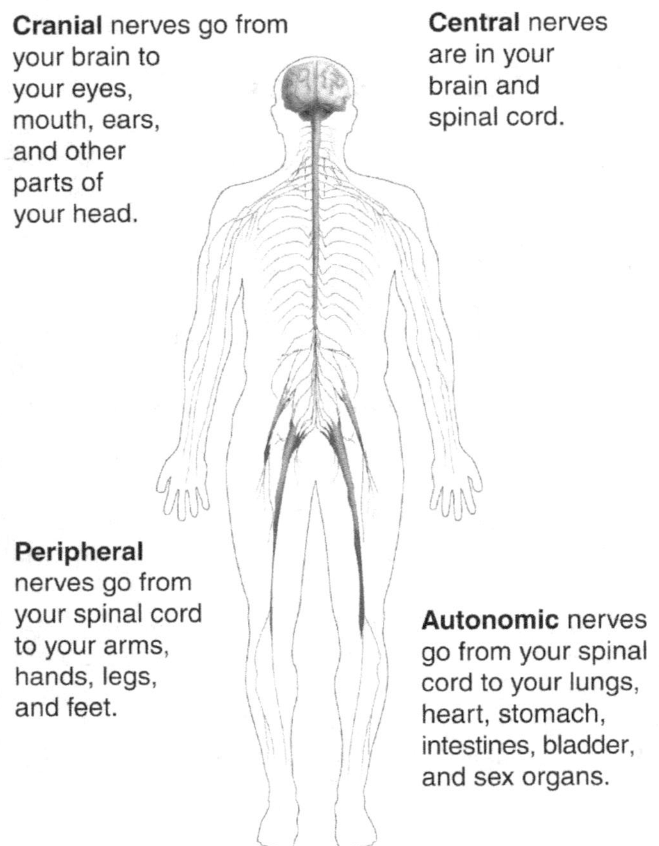

1. The Central Nervous System (CNS)

The brain is the centre of the CNS, which receives impulses/sensations that are interpreted and stored in the mind. Our memory is based on the accumulation of these stored impulses. The brain receives and transmits impulses via the nerves to various parts of the body.

The main parts of the brain are as follows:

A. The Cerebrum

The cerebrum forms the bulk of the brain and is supported on the brain stem. It is divided into a right hemisphere (which controls the left side of the body) and a left hemisphere (which controls the right side of the body).

The cerebrum performs the following functions:

- Receiving sensory stimuli and conveying them to the consciousness
- Initiating all voluntary movements
- Retaining received impulses as a part of our memory
- Formulating ideas; i.e. intelligence
- Exercising control over some of the bodily functions
- Exercising control of the lower parts of the brain

B. The Hypothalamus

This is the lower part of the fore brain and helps to control the cardiovascular and respiratory systems, food intake and digestion, sex and maternal instincts, and emotions.

It is closely linked to the ANS, and the involuntary and voluntary functions of the body.

C. The Cerebellum

Known as the lesser brain, it performs the following functions:

- Helping to maintain muscular tone
- Coordinating muscular movement
- Receiving impulses from the ears, joints and muscles to maintain balance and equilibrium
- Memorising complicated movements from experience

D. The Brain Stem

This consists of the mid-brain (which transmits impulses from the two hemispheres), the pons Varolii (which transmits impulses to and from the cerebrum) and the medulla oblangata (which connects other parts of the brain to the spinal cord). The medulla oblangata also contains vital centres such as the respiratory centre, vasomotor centre (for the regulation of the heartbeat) and the centre affecting some of the digestive functions.

2. The Peripheral Nervous System (PNS)

The spinal cord is a continuation of the medulla oblangata, and runs inside and is protected by the vertebral column (back bone). It provides the main pathway for the nerves and is the source for 31 pairs of nerves, which form the PNS.

The PNS provides the connection between the internal or external stimuli and the CNS to allow the body to respond to its environment.

The nerves in the PNS connect the CNS to the sensory organs, such as the eye and ear, and to other organs of the body, muscles, blood vessels and glands.

The following diagram shows the nerves of the PNS:

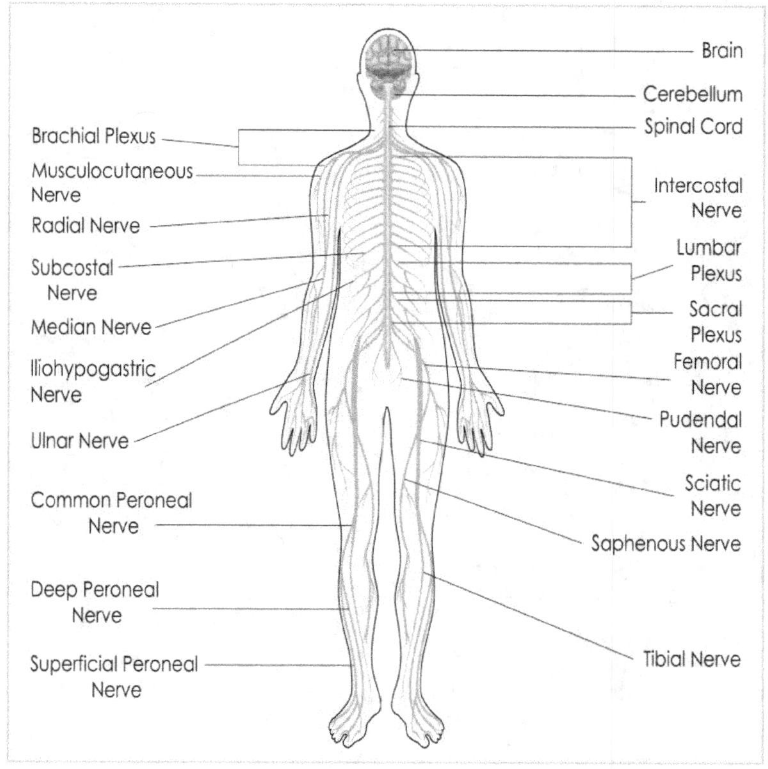

3. The Autonomic (or Involuntary) Nervous System (ANS)

The ANS exercises its functions independently of the CNS, but they are closely related and interact with each other. Its two parts, the sympathetic and parasympathetic nervous systems control the functioning of the internal organs, and perform the functions to stimulate or restrict as described in the previous diagram.

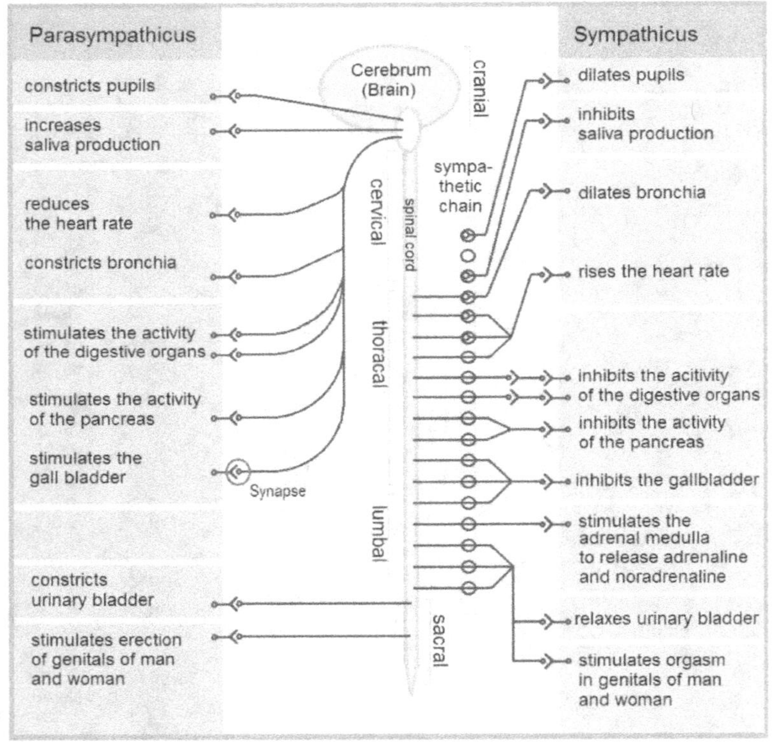
Parasympathicus
Sympathicus
constricts pupils
increases
saliva production
reduces
the heart rate
constricts bronchia
stimulates the activity
of the digestive organs
stimulates the activity
of the pancreas
stimulates the
gall bladder
Synapse
constricts
urinary bladder
stimulates erection
of genitals of man
and woman
Cerebrum
(Brain)
cranial
sympa-
thetic
chain
cervical
spinal cord
thoracal
lumbal
sacral
dilates pupils
inhibits
saliva production
dilates bronchia
rises the heart rate
inhibits the acitivity
of the digestive organs
inhibits the activity
of the pancreas
inhibits the gallbladder
stimulates the
adrenal medulla
to release adrenaline
and noradrenaline
relaxes urinary bladder
stimulates orgasm
in genitals of man
and woman

E. THE MUSCULAR SYSTEM

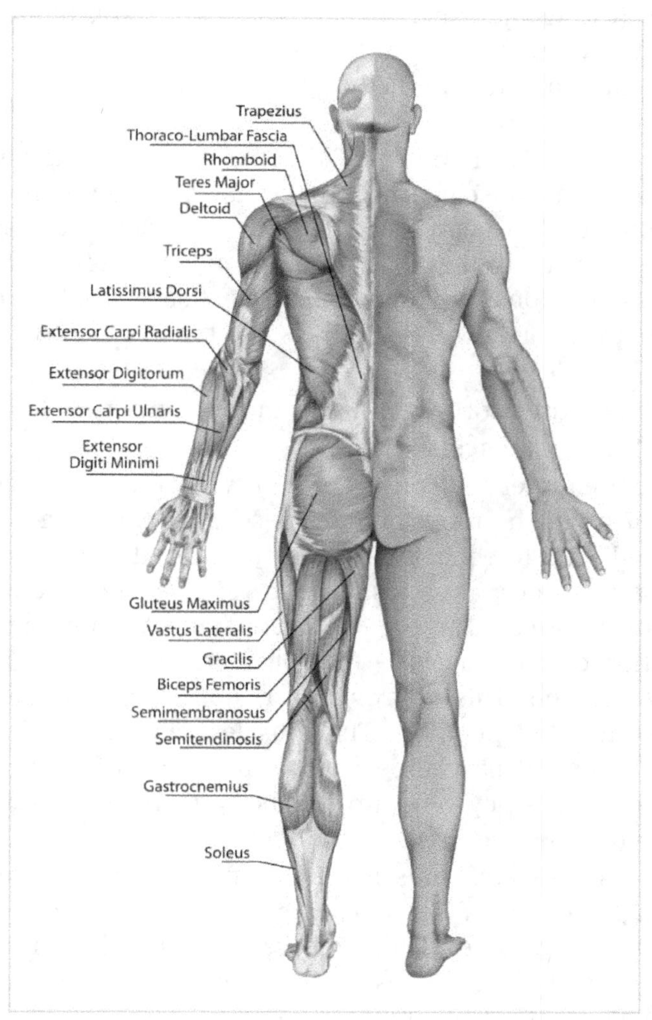

The **muscular system** is responsible for the following vital functions:
1) Providing movement to the parts of the body.
2) Providing movement to substances – food, blood and energy – within the body.
3) Generating heat in the body.

Attached to the bones of the skeletal system are about 700 named muscles that make up roughly half of a person's body weight. Each of these muscles is a discrete organ constructed from skeletal muscle tissue, blood vessels, tendons and nerves. Muscle tissue is also found inside the heart, digestive organs and blood vessels.

There are three sorts of muscles in the body, as follows:
1. Voluntary Muscles
These are under the control of your will and are concerned primarily with movement. These muscles are called 'striped' due to their microscopic appearance and include the respiratory muscles, which are 'striped' but are automatic. Related to the function of movement is another function of the muscles – that of maintaining posture and body position. This is provided by holding the muscles in the contracted position. The muscles responsible for the body's posture have the greatest endurance of all muscles in the body—they hold up the body throughout the day without becoming tired.

Most skeletal muscles are attached to two bones, through tendons. Tendons are tough bands of dense regular connective tissue whose strong collagen fibres firmly attach the muscles to the bones. Tendons are under extreme stress when muscles pull on them, so they are very strong, and are woven into the coverings of both muscles and bones.

Muscles move by shortening their length, pulling on tendons and moving bones closer to each other. One of the bones is pulled towards the other bone, which remains stationary. The place on the stationary bone that is connected to the muscle via tendons is called the origin. The place on the moving bone that is connected to the muscle via tendons is called the insertion. The belly of the muscle is the fleshy part of the muscle in between the tendons that does the actual contraction. Most muscles have an opposite number (antagonist); e.g. the biceps at the front of the upper arm contracts to bend the forearm and its opposite muscle at the back of the forearm, the triceps, straightens the forearm when it contracts. To contract, a muscle receives an electrical message along the nerve that causes the chemical change leading to contraction.

The final function of muscle tissue is the generation of body heat. As a result of the high metabolic rate of the contracting muscle, our muscular system produces a great deal of waste heat. Many small muscle contractions within the body produce our natural body heat. When we exert ourselves more than normal, the extra muscle contractions lead to a rise in body temperature and eventually to sweating.

2. Involuntary Muscles

These muscles are under the control of the ANS. These muscles are called 'unstriped' but the 'unstriped' muscles of bladder are under learned voluntary control.

Involuntary muscles are found in the stomach, intestines, arteries, tubes of the lungs, uterus and other organs.

Unlike voluntary muscles, these muscles contract slowly and rhythmically, and are under the control of the ANS.

3. Cardiac Muscles

These are found in the heart and are striped with interconnections. The muscle of the heart is a special form of involuntary muscle. It is not under the control of the will but has the form of a strip of colour resembling that seen in striped muscles. It has the special property of automatic rhythmic contraction, which can occur independently of its nerve supply.

F. THE CIRCULATORY SYSTEM

The main function of the circulatory system is to supply oxygen and nourishment to every tissue and organ in the body, and remove the waste products resulting from their activities.

Pranayamas and yogic *asanas* can help to improve the health and efficient functioning of the organs of our circulatory system.

The essential components of the circulatory system are the heart, blood and blood vessels.

1. The Heart

The heart is a muscular pump that lies in the chest (thorax) between the two lungs and above the surface of the diaphragm. It is located behind the breast bone and extends to the left of our body.

The heart is divided into a right and a left partition, each of which is further split into an upper and lower chamber. The upper thin walled chamber is known as the auricle (or atrium) and is the receiving chamber for the blood, and the lower thick-walled chamber, known as the ventricle, is the one that distributes the blood out. There is a protecting valve between the two chambers allowing the blood to flow only from the auricle to the ventricle.

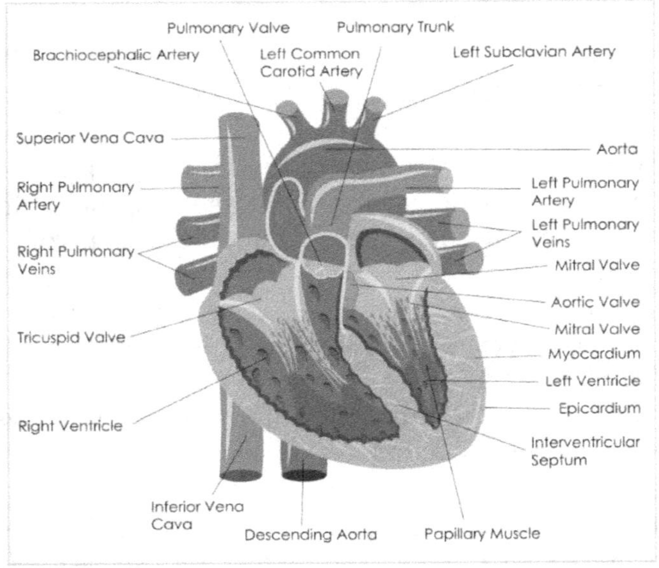

De-oxygenated blood is collected from various parts of the body and is passed into the right auricle via the large veins: the superior and inferior vena cava. Moving down through the valve, it passes into the right ventricle and leaves the heart by the pulmonary artery.

The blood is then transported to the lungs via the pulmonary arteries, where it is re-oxygenated and taken back to the left auricle by the four pulmonary veins. Passing down through the valve to the left ventricle, the blood leaves the heart by the main artery of the body, the aorta.

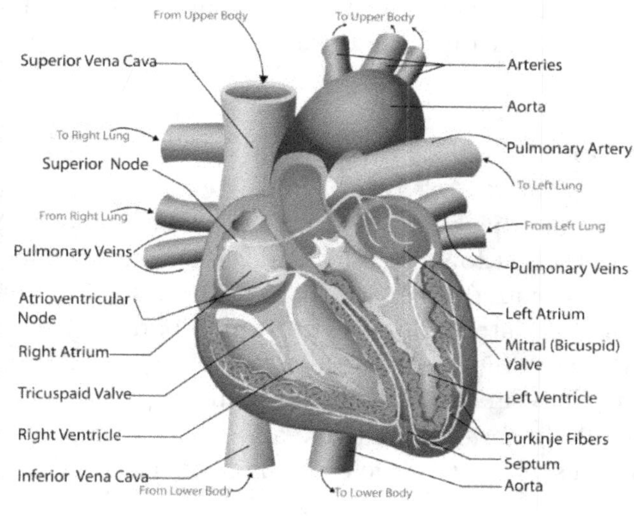

The heart has its own generator, which sends out electrical pulses and produces rhythmic contractions known as heartbeats.

2. The Arteries

These are thick-walled, elastic, muscular tubes whose function is to take the blood away from the heart into a network of capillaries. Pressure created by the heart pump enables the arteries to pulsate and maintain the forwards flow of the blood. Due to the high oxygen content, the pigment haemoglobin makes the blood in the arteries red in colour (except in the pulmonary artery).

3. The Capillaries

These are minute hair-like blood vessels that connect the arteries and veins. The interchange of oxygen, nourishment and waste products takes place between the blood and tissue cells through the walls of the capillaries. These provide a dense and vast network throughout the body.

4. The Veins

Veins take blood back from the tissues to the heart, for it to be pumped back to the lungs for re-oxygenation. Veins contain blood at low pressure and rely on the compression of muscles around them, gravity and the valves (in some of the veins) to stop the backflow of blood in the wrong direction. Having given up its oxygen to the tissues, the blood in the veins turns blueish red in colour.

Smaller arteries (arterioles) and smaller veins (venules) have nerves which provide control on their actions.

5. The Blood

The key functions of the blood are as follows:

1) Carrying oxygen to the tissues by means of haemoglobin in the red cells.
2) Removing waste products from the tissues – carbon dioxide is carried to the lungs, and urea is carried to the kidneys, lungs and skin where the excess is removed.
3) Carrying water, nourishment and other substances taken by mouth to all parts of the body, as needed.
4) Carrying hormones and other chemical messengers.
5) Carrying antibodies to agents and preventing disease.
6) Aiding the defence mechanism of the body through the white cells.
7) Carrying heat from heat producing organs.
8) Washing out and sealing a wounded area by clotting.

⸺ ✳ ⸺

7. References and Acknowledgements

ACKNOWLEDGEMENTS

I would like to express my gratitude to:

- Gill Pendreich my yoga teacher for her guidance and advice on the chapter on the practice

- Dr Madan Mohan Lal, orthopaedic surgeon for his guidance on the medical aspects of the practice

- Samani Dr Pratibha Pragya for her valuable input and comments

- Lindsay Corten of Corten Editorial for providing proofreading and editorial service

- My daughter Sasha for her input on number of iterations of the book

- Last but not least, my wife for her unstinting support during my writing of this book

REFERENCES

✓ Google and Wikipedia for extensive research on all aspects of the book

✓ Brown, Christina (2017). *The Modern Yoga Bible.* London, UK: Godsfield Press

✓ Giovanni (2015). *Types of Meditation – An Overview of 23 Meditation Techniques.* Live and Dare [online] Available at: https://liveanddare.com/types-of-meditation

✓ Hewitt, James (1992). The Complete Yoga Book. London, UK: Rider

✓ Iyengar, B.K.S. (2015). *Light on Yoga.* New York, NY: Harper Thorsons.

✓ Macey, Ashley (2017). *How Yoga and Meditation Can Biologically Reverse Stress.* [online] Available at: https://www.brit.co/yoga-and-meditation-can-biologically-reverse-stress/

✓ Macey, Ashley (YYYY). *Article name.* Frontiers in Immunology. [online] Available at: website

✓ McCall MD, Timothy (2007). 38 Health Benefits of Yoga, Yoga Journal, [online] Available at: https://www.yogajournal.com/lifestyle/count-yoga-38-ways-yoga-keeps-fit

✓ Muktibodhananda, Swami Saraswati (1998). Light on Hatha Yoga. Hatha Yoga Pradipika. Munger, India: Bihar School of Yoga.

✓ National Institute of Diabetes and Digestive and Kidney Diseases (YYYY). Photo of Nervous System and Digestive System. National Institutes of Health. [online] Available at:

✓ Ornish, Dr Dean (1997). *Program for Reversing Heart Disease*, United States: Ivy Books

✓ Shannahoff-Khalsa, David S. (2007). Kundalini Yoga Meditation. London, UK: W. W. Norton & Company

✓ *The Guardian*'s Science Weekly

✓ Token Rock (n.d.). *Chakras*. [online] Available at: https://www.tokenrock.com

✓ Tobler, Albert and Herrmann, Susan (2013). *The Rough Guide to Mindfulness*. London, UK: Penguin Books

✓ Yoga in Daily Life (n.d.). [online] Available at: https://www.yogaindailylife.org

✓ Yoga in Daily Life (n.d.). *The Full Yoga Breath*. [online] Available at: https://www.yogaindailylife.org

8. Glossary of Terms

Sanskrit and other terms	Meaning
Abhijna	Transcendental powers
Ahimsa	Non-violence
Ajna chakra	The *chakra* located at the eyebrow centre, also known as the 'third eye' (also see '*chakra*' entry)
Anahata chakra	The *chakra* based at the heart centre
Anapana sati	Mindfulness of breathing
Anulom vilom pranayama	Breathing technique to balance the flow of breath between the two sides of the body
Anusara yoga	A form of yoga developed by American yogi John Friend
Aparigraha	Non-possessiveness or non-attachment
Asana	'seat' in Sanskrit, but commonly used to refer to postures
Ashoka	Indian emperor who ruled India around 260 BC; he became a follower of Jainism but later

converted to Buddhism

Ashtanga	Eight limbs or eight-fold
Asteya	Non-stealing
Atma	Soul
Aum, ham, arham, yam, ram, lam	Words/sounds used in mantra meditation
B.K.S. Iyengar	Founder of the form of yoga named after him: Iyengar Yoga
Bahya pranayama	Holding the breath out
Bhakti yoga	Path of devotion and worship – one of the paths of yoga
Bhramari pranayama	*'bhramari'* means 'honeybee' in Sanskrit; this pranayama is used for calming the mind and help one connect with one's inner self
Bhujangasana	Cobra pose
Bikram yoga	A form of yoga founded by Bikram Choudhury
Brahamcharya	Celibacy
Bridge pose	'bridge' translates to *'setu-bandha'* in Sanskrit; this pose is traditionally called *'setubandhasana'*
British Wheel of Yoga	British national yoga organisation
Buddha	Gautama Buddha, who was the

	ascetic on whose teachings Buddhism was founded
Buddhist	Pertaining to Buddhism
Cat pose	'cat' translates to *'marjari'* in Sanskrit; this pose is traditionally called *'marjariasana'*
Chakra	Means 'wheel' in Sanskrit; these are subtle energy centres in the human body, of which there are seven
Chitta	Consciousness
Dharna	Concentration
Dhyana	Meditation (the second stage of the progressive states of meditation – *dharna, dhyana* and *samadhi)*
Dog pose	'dog' translates to *'shvan'* in Sanskrit; this pose is traditionally called *'shvnasana'*
Enlightenment	The state of having knowledge or understanding; in Indian philosophy it is the 'highest spiritual state'
Full yoga breath	Abdominal breathing utilising the maximum capacity of the lungs
S.N. Goenka	Burmese-Indian teacher of *vipassana* meditation
Gyan mudra	A hand position in which tips of the first finger and thumbs are brought together

Hatha yoga	An old system that includes most styles of yoga, and includes the practice of *asanas* and *pranayamas*
Hatha yoga pradipika	A treatise on Hatha Yoga by Swami Muktibodhananda
Ida and *pingla*	The twin energy channels that criss-cross at the *chakras* and run from the *muladhara chakra*, go all the way up to *sahasrara*, and, finally, end at the left and right nostrils, respectively
International Day of Yoga	A day to celebrate and promote yoga worldwide
Ishvar-pranidhan	Contemplation of the supreme being (God)
Iyengar yoga	A form of Hatha Yoga developed by B.K.S. Iyengar
Jainism	The religion founded by Lord Mahavira, and known for its core tenets of 'ahimsa' (non-violence), 'aparigraha' (non-attachment) and 'anekantvad' (multiplicity of truth)
Japa	The repeated chanting of a sacred sound (word)
Jnana yoga	The path of wisdom – one of the paths of yoga
Kapalbhati pranayama	A pranayama that oxygenates the body and improves circulation

Karma yoga	The path of action – one of the paths of yoga
Katha upnishad	An Indian scripture
Kriya	Sanskrit word meaning 'action'
Kundalini	It is the name of the *chakra* at the base of the spine and also refers to the dormant spiritual energy in our body
Locust pose	'locust' translates to '*shalabha*' in Sanskrit; this pose is traditionally called '*shalabhasana*'
Mahavira	An enlightened soul and the founder of Jainism
Manipura chakra	The *chakra* based at the navel centre
Mantra	A word(s) or group of words used for chanting
Meditation	A practice that enables one to concentrate on one object to the exclusion of all others
Mindfulness	Contemplation – the process of bringing one's attention to the experiences occurring at the present moment
Moksha	'Liberation' from the cycle of death and re-birth; salvation
Mudra	The positioning of the hands
Muladhara chakra	The 'root' *chakra* at the base of the spine

Nadi	Sanskrit meaning 'stream'; the channels through which subtle energy or *prana* flows in our body
Namaste	Indian greeting with the palms of the hands held together in front of the chest
Nirvana	A state of enlightenment; a place of perfect peace and happiness
Niyama	Observance
Patanjali	The Indian sage who developed the eight-fold path called the *Sutras of Patanjali*
Prana	Life force
Pranayama	The control of the breath
Preksha	Seeing things as they are
Qi (chi)	Life energy
Qi gong (chi kung)	The cultivation of life energy
Raja yoga	The path of the control of the mind – one of the paths of yoga
Respiratory system	Consists of the series of organs responsible for taking in oxygen and expelling carbon dioxide from the body
Sahasrara chakra	The *chakra* located at the top of the head, which connects us with the divine source/energy; '*sahasrara*' in Sanskrit means thousand petaled

Samadhi	A state of intense concentration achieved through meditation -the final step in the *Yoga Sutras*
Samatha	Equanimity
Santosha	Contentment
Sati	Mindfulness
Satya	Truth
Shaucha	Cleanliness
Shavasana	*'shava'* in Sanskrit means 'corpse' – it refers to the corpse pose
Shikantza	Means 'just sitting'
Sivanada yoga	A form of gentle yoga developed by Swami Sivananda
Spinal twist	Creating a gentle twist in the spine by holding the shoulders in one place and gently turning the pelvis
Spondylitis	A type of arthritis affecting the spine
Sukhasana	Cross-legged sitting posture in yoga
Surya namaskar	The sun salutation – a sequence of postures
Sushmana nadi	The main energy channels that run from the *mooladhara chakra* at the base and all the way up to the *sahasrara chakra*
Svadhistana chakra	The *chakra* based in the lower abdominal area

Swadhyaya	Self-study; however, it is also interpreted as a study of religious books/scriptures
Swami ramdev	21st-century Indian yogi who has created a resurgence of yoga in India
Tao	Means 'nature' in Chinese
Tao te ching	A Chinese philosopher
Taoist	Pertaining to Tao philosophy
Tapas	Persistent meditation
Theologian	A person who studies religious faith
Third eye	The point on the forehead at the centre of the eyes; the position of the *ajna chakra*
Tirthankara	An enlightened soul
Transcendental	Relating to a spiritual realm
Trataka	Staring at a single point
Vajrasana	'*vajra*' means 'thunderbolt' in Sanskrit; the posture in which a person sits upright in a kneeling position
Vipassana	'Seeing things as they really are'
Vishuddhi chakra	The *chakra* based at the bottom of the throat
We-wei	Means 'non-action or action without the influence of its outcome' in Chinese
Yama	Abstinence
Yoga	The union of body and mind

Yoga nidra	A state of relaxation where the body is in a state of sleep, but the mind is alert
Yoga sutras	The eight-fold path of yoga founded by sage Patanjali
Zen	The school of Mahayana Buddhism that originated in China

9 781721 712588